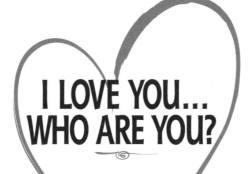

I LOVE YOU...
WHO ARE YOU?

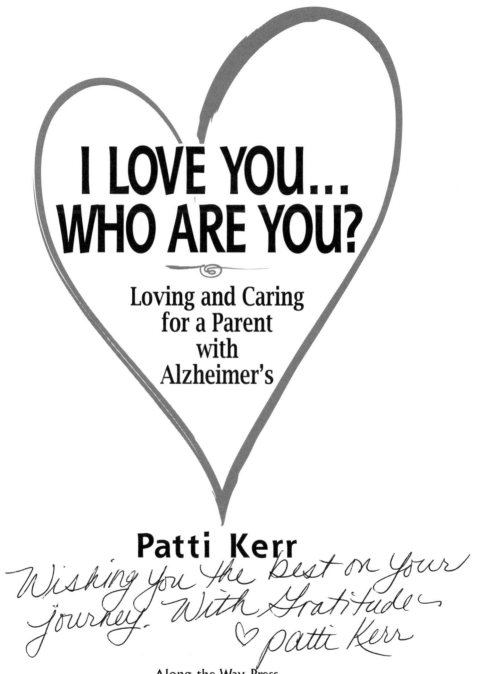

I LOVE YOU...
WHO ARE YOU?

Loving and Caring
for a Parent
with
Alzheimer's

Patti Kerr

Wishing you the best on your journey. With Gratitude ♡ patti kerr

Along the Way Press

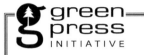

I LOVE YOU...WHO ARE YOU? Loving and Caring for a Parent with Alzheimer's
Copyright © 2010 by Patti Kerr

Along the Way Press
PO Box 2443
Flemington, NJ 08822-1437

Cover Design: James Lebbad
Editor: Joy E. Stocke
Interior Design: Sans Serif, Inc.

ISBN: 978-0-9845989-9-1
Library of Congress Control Number: 2010914872

Ordering Information:
Additional copies can be ordered directly from the author's website: www.pattikerr.com. Special discounts are available on quantity purchases by corporations, associations, and others. For details, contact the publisher at the address above.

Printed in the United States of America on recycled acid-free paper using nontoxic soy-based ink.

To my mother and father
and to everyone who has,
or will one day,
love and care
for a parent with
Alzheimer's.

CONTENTS

ACKNOWLEDGEMENTS

In 1988, I wrote "My Life List:" Seventy-two things I'd like to accomplish in the time I'm given on Earth. *"Write a book"* was #21 on the list. But I had no idea how much writing a book — this book — would change me.

I have been blessed with an abundance of people who joined me on this journey and who freely and generously offered their wisdom, insight and support. I owe them my deepest, and heartfelt, gratitude.

To those who shared their lives and struggles as well as their experience and expertise, I thank you for your courage, your honesty and the enormity of love in your hearts: Shirley S. Albright, Kitty C. Allen, Jeffrey A. Asher, Esq., Charlie Athanas, Heather Barbod, Sue Barna, David Bartholomew, Shelly Beach, Victoria A. Beckner, Jaye Bird, Cheryl Reilly Bishop, Kristen Blankenship Mueller, J. Lucy Boyd RN/BSN, Karen Boyd, Roberta Brassard, Alan Bryant, Jerry Buck, Karen Bump, Diane Carbo RN, Rebecca Ciurczak, Grace Clifton, Peggy Collinsmith, Alissa and Tom Cotter, William T. Crum, Kelly Duerr, Karen Drucker, Mike Dufford, Sean Dufford, Gayle Erickson, Marie Fostino, Betsy S. Franz, Donna G., Leslie Anne Galloway, Sandie Glass, B. Lynn Goodwin, Rev. Cynthia Greb, Kristina Greco, Susan R. Grossman, Dorothy Harper, Jennifer Hicks, Patricia C. Hilton, Wanda Jewell, Mary L. Kehrer, Jeannot Kensinger, Rhonda-Lee Kensinger, Sabrina G. Kensinger, Bryan Kerr, Devon Kerr Cady, Jeanne Kessler, Ninah Kessler LCSW, Dan Koffman, Frank Lee, Joyce Leftly, Lois M. Lewis, Cassie Lohrum, Janice Sutphin Lowstuter, Debra Madonna, Bonnie F. Malone, Dorothy Malone, Deborah Meredith LRT/CTRS, Tracy Mobley, Judy Morgan, Mary E. Murphy, Barbara Nechacov, N.E.W. Curative Rehabilitation, Inc., Chris Nutter, Patricia Fares-O'Malley, PhD, Carole Pepe, Mary S., Lynn Shaw MSW/LCSW, Ami Simms, Jennie Simms, Pat Reilly Skinner, Allison Snow, Joy St.John Johnson, Steven M. Sultanoff, PhD, Ann Thomas, Connie V. & Carmen, Max Wallack, Kathie Watkins.

To my parents, Joe and Penny Kerr. Thank you for being a real-life example of true love and for giving my sons and me a lifetime of love. Your love, guidance and support allowed me to live the majority of my days on the sunny side of life. I love you more than you will ever know.

To my sons, Mike and Sean. Thank you for everything — for being there through it all and for your love, encouragement and support. You have hearts so large and wise that I am forever honored to be your mother. I love you — always have, always will.

To Joe, Kelly, Devon and Bryan. I am blessed to call you my family — and to be part of a family that cares so deeply for one another.

To Robb. Thank you for believing in me — and this book — and for your love through the years.

To Brooke, my precious puppy. Thank you for sleeping peacefully next to me as I wrote and for being my faithful, loving companion on this journey.

To the Five Wise Women: Sue Barna, Diane J. Clark, Melanie E. Martin, Judy Thorne Morgan and Kerri Schmatz. Thank you, ladies, for the time, energy, dedication and love you poured into this book — and me. I am so grateful to have each of you in my life.

To my bounty of friends, the Queen's Court, my Goddess Sisters, the Writers Coffeehouse, the Liars Club, and everyone at Basil Bandwagon Natural Market. I wish I could list you all individually by name. Thank you for being there through the years I helped care for my mother and as I wrote this book. Thank you for the cups of coffee, e-mails, hugs, laughter, love, tears and encouragement. You were the wind beneath my wings more times than you will ever know.

To Bernice. At the end of my mother's journey, you loved and cared for her as if she were your own. Thank you. You are my sister for life.

To Hunterdon Hospice. Thank you for making the end of my mother's journey peaceful and graceful and for teaching me how to let go with love.

To Jonathan Maberry. Thank you for guiding me to — and along — the writing path. You are a brilliant author, mentor, teacher and friend.

To Joy E. Stocke, Editor Extraordinaire. You are a woman of amazing insight and incredible wisdom. Your belief in this project helped shape this book — and me — into something I once only dreamed of. I am forever grateful I had you by my side on this journey and am blessed to call you my friend.

To Karen Drucker. Your music allowed my mother and me to stay connected and communicate with one another at the end of her journey — and beyond. You, and your music, are a blessing to the world.

I am so blessed.

PROLOGUE

"I Love You...Who Are You?"

I was wiping my kitchen counter when I heard a knock at the front door. I opened the door and saw my mother standing there, looking panicked and afraid.

"Mama, what's wrong?" I said.

She walked into my living room and held out her hands, pointing at her fingernails. "Look. Look," she said as she began to cry.

I looked at her hands and fingernails. They both looked fine, healthy.

"What's wrong with them?" my mother asked, tears now streaming down her face.

I took hold of her hands and looked again. And then I realized. Putting my arm around my mother's shoulder, I led her over to the couch. As we sat down, I began to explain. "Mama, it's okay. Everything is okay. There's nothing wrong, Mama. Nothing at all."

"Really?" she said.

"Really, Mama. You had cancer and the medicine they gave you made you lose your fingernails. But now the cancer is gone. So these," I said, pointing at her fingers, "are your fingernails. They're growing back and that's a good thing. It means you're healthy."

"Really?" she asked again.

"I promise," I said, giving her a reassuring hug.

My mother smiled, relaxed, and asked me what I'd been doing — not remembering we'd just spent the entire day together. Then she looked at her fingernails again. For a second, I was afraid she'd forget what we just talked about. But instead, she smiled, saying, "Look how long they are."

"They *are* long, Mama, long and beautiful. Would you like a manicure?"

"Sure," she said.

Despite all she had forgotten, my mother still remembered — and enjoyed — manicures. I was grateful because it was one small thing I could still do with (and for) her. I cherished these small blessings, snippets of time, and sacred moments.

As I filed her nails, we continued to talk and laugh. Then, as I was putting the finishing touches on her last nail, my mother looked into my eyes, smiled, and in the sweetest, gentlest voice said, "You are always so nice to me."

I smiled, my heart melting. My mother continued, "I love you."

I opened my mouth to tell her I loved her too but, before I could utter a word, she finished her sentence.

"Who are you?"

Our Journey with Alzheimer's

Our family's journey with Alzheimer's began with my grand-mother, Catherine Wytak Sahaydak.

Born in the Ukraine, Kate (as she was called by family and friends) left her family while still a young woman and boarded a boat to head across the ocean for America. There she met and married Hnat Sahaydak, a fellow Ukrainian, and together they moved from New York City to rural New Jersey. They bought a small farm and raised chickens, vegetables and six children — four boys and two girls. In 1959, at the age of 62, her beloved Hnat died from cancer. My grandmother was devastated.

Since we lived three blocks from my grandmother, my mother and I visited her every day. Most Saturday nights my cousin Linda and I stayed overnight at my grandmother's house. Together, we'd watch *The Lawrence Welk Show* and then crawl into my grandmother's massive featherbed. After saying our prayers together, my grandmother would continue praying alone in Ukrainian, beating her chest with her fist and sobbing. My cousin and I didn't understand her words but we knew she was crying for our grandfather. Despite filling her days with family, friends, gardening and cooking, my grandmother never got over the loss of her beloved Hnat.

My grandmother stood 4 feet 8 inches tall but was, as she often told me, "strong as a bull" — both physically and mentally.

However, a few years after I graduated from high school, she began having minor bouts of forgetfulness. My mother took her to the doctor who said forgetfulness was a normal part of aging. When the forgetfulness became more severe, my mother took my grandmother back to the doctor. This time he said my grandmother had "hardening of the arteries in her brain" and that there was nothing he (or anyone) could do to cure or help her.

My mother immediately called a meeting of her brothers and sister. Since they all agreed that my grandmother should remain in her home, my mother prepared a schedule, dividing the week into manageable chunks for each of them to watch over and care for her. For a time, all went well and it seemed the family had found a workable solution.

Every morning, my grandmother walked to the A&P grocery store one block away to buy bread or milk. The managers and clerks, who all knew her by name, began calling my mother to tell her they were concerned about my grandmother because they often saw her wandering aimlessly after leaving their store. Even though the staff always made sure my grandmother got home safely, my mother's concerns for my grandmother's continued safety grew. She realized her mother who, as a young woman had journeyed alone across an ocean to a new country, was now having trouble finding her way home from the store just one block away.

The doctors listened to my mother's concerns and continued to write prescription after prescription to try and relieve my grandmother's ever-changing symptoms. Soon my grandmother had an arsenal of pharmaceuticals to address the agitation, sleeplessness, confusion, hallucinations, anger and other emotions that now filled her life and mind.

As my grandmother's behavior grew more erratic and unpredictable, so did the caregiving. Family members suddenly had "conflicts" and asked to be removed from the schedule. Others gave no warning and simply didn't show up for their designated time slot. Large gaps began to appear in the schedule — gaps when my grandmother was being left alone.

Like my grandmother, my mother was mentally and physically strong. That, along with her endless energy and amazing organizational skills, served her well as she continued to handle our family's — and now my grandmother's — life with apparent ease. On her way home from work, my mother stopped to see my grandmother and, since she often found her alone, my mother began spending nights at my grandmother's house. In the morning, she would feed my grandmother before heading off to work. During the day, she would call my grandmother to make sure someone was with her and that she was safe. For a while, all was fine and my mother was able to keep up the pace. And then my grandmother entered yet another phase.

In this new phase, my grandmother would grow agitated in the late afternoon. Often, by the time my mother arrived after work, my grandmother would be pacing and angry. At night, my grandmother wandered around the house or tried climbing out the windows to escape the people and things she now saw lurking in her home. The doctors added more medication to try and relieve the new symptoms. Sometimes the medications worked — most nights they didn't.

My mother was getting little (if any) sleep. In the morning, she faced the difficult decision of going to work and possibly leaving my grandmother alone or taking another unpaid day off from work. My mother was now working, most days, around the clock without a break. As my mother grew increasingly tired, my father grew increasingly concerned.

One evening my mother phoned my father, in tears. My grandmother was having another sleepless night. My mother was exhausted and couldn't remember when, or if, she'd given my grandmother her medication. Knowing my grandmother could become violent or difficult to handle if she missed a dosage, my mother was also afraid if she'd already given her the medication, she ran the risk of overmedicating my grandmother.

"I don't know what to do," my mother cried into the phone.

My father knew exactly what to do. He called another family meeting.

♡

Despite my mother's desire to continue caring for her mother at home, the family decided it was time to put my grandmother into a nursing home. My mother begged her family to reconsider, but they remained steadfast. My grandmother's house was sold and she was moved into the first nursing home that had an available bed. My mother was crushed, defeated and distraught.

To add to my mother's distress, my grandmother cried and begged my mother every time she visited to take her home.

"Please," my grandmother cried, rattling the side rails of her bed. "Take me home. Let's go. I want to go home."

Slowly, over time, those requests lessened and eventually vanished — along with my grandmother's memories of the people and places she loved.

♡

My mother remained involved in my grandmother's care. She did her laundry and washed and styled her hair. She cooked my grandmother's favorite foods and would sit at the nursing home and feed her. When it became obvious my grandmother wasn't receiving adequate care, my mother moved her from facility to facility until she finally found a wonderful, caring place that treated my grandmother with the dignity, respect and love she so richly deserved.

Despite my mother's unconditional love and constant care, my grandmother continued to vanish day-after-day and minute-by-minute behind the veil of Alzheimer's.

♡

It was becoming more and more difficult for me to visit my grandmother. Most of the time, she lay in her bed completely unresponsive and unaware that I, or anyone, was in the room. Nonetheless, one Christmas morning, I went with my mom to visit her. As we entered the room, I could see my grandmother staring vacantly into space. Mom and I kissed her, but she remained unresponsive.

As my mother fed her breakfast, I decided to venture out on a limb. "Do you know what today is, Granny?" I asked.

"Sure," she said in her adorable Ukrainian accent.

"You do?" I asked, stunned that she had responded to my question.

"Sure. It's Christmas."

"And do you know who comes today?"

"Sure," she said again. "Santa Claus."

Still floored, I kept going. "And do you think Santa will bring you anything?"

"Sure," she said, smiling, "Why not? I've been a good girl."

We laughed as I wrapped my arms around my grandmother and gave her a hug and kiss. "Yes, you have been a good girl. Merry Christmas, Granny. I love you."

She looked into my eyes — and then she was gone. Back into the void, her eyes staring vacantly into space.

That short conversation with my grandmother was one of the greatest Christmas gifts I ever received. It also taught me a very important lesson about Alzheimer's. I realized in those few minutes that, even when it appeared the disease had taken away my grandmother's ability to understand and respond to others, she was still "in there."

After that, every time I visited my grandmother, even though she didn't respond, I talked to her as if she were fully present. I talked about things we had done together through the years and told her about my life now. And I always made sure I told her how much I loved her.

The conversation we had on Christmas morning was the last one we ever had. A few months later, my grandmother died.

♡

After my grandmother's death, my parents promised one another that, should either of them get sick, they would always care for one another at home and would never put the other into a nursing home or facility. Even though my mother knew my grandmother had been well cared for, she never forgot or forgave herself that she hadn't cared for her mother at home.

Whenever my mother talked about my grandmother, she said she wished she'd been able to do more for her — and that no one in our family would ever fall prey to the disease.

Over time, we returned to our everyday lives and put Alzheimer's back on the shelf and out of our minds.

And then, in September 2003, it returned.

♡

"The mini-mental status test clearly demonstrated impairment in the range of a mild dementia. It is likely your mother has early Alzheimer's disease."

I put the letter down on the table, numb. I, as well as my father and brother, had suspected something was wrong since the summer of 2001 when Mom had a minor auto accident. No one had been injured and her car only sustained minor damage but Mom talked and cried about the accident constantly. Following the 9/11 attack on the World Trade Center, despite the horror and tragedy unfolding on the television, she continued to only talk about the car accident.

Next, she began to repeat things, misplaced items, and forget people's names. What was equally striking, and upsetting, was that my mother, who had always loved to drive, never got behind the wheel of a car again.

As Mom's behavior and personality continued to slowly and subtly change, our concerns and suspicions grew. Yet, despite the obvious signs, my father, brother and I chose to believe it was normal forgetfulness. After all, who doesn't repeat themselves, forget someone's name, or misplace their wallet or keys?

Now, as I picked up the letter and read those nine words: *"It is likely your mother has early Alzheimer's disease,"* the doctor confirmed our suspicions — and changed our world.

Those nine words, turned my mother's biggest fear — that she might one day succumb to the same disease, and fate, as her mother — into a reality and forced me to face the reality that one day my mother, my best friend, the woman who had given me the gift of life, might one day forget my name and who I was.

♡

The doctor gave my mother samples of, and wrote a prescription for, Aricept. He explained it was a relatively new medication that could potentially slow down memory loss. My mother didn't say a word.

On the drive home, my mother still didn't say a word. Once home, she walked into the bathroom and flushed the samples down the toilet. She then walked into the kitchen, ripped up the prescription and told my father, "There is nothing wrong with my brain!"

I asked my father what we were going to do.

"Nothing," he said.

Having watched my grandmother's journey with Alzheimer's, my father reasoned that if my mother knew she was facing the same fate, she couldn't bear it. He asked my brother and me not to talk about it or discuss it with my mother.

"If she knows, it will kill her," he said.

So we remained silent. No one said a word and we pretended nothing had happened. For a while, it worked. Mom went about her day with only minor bouts of forgetfulness. We heard the same story or answered the same question more often in the course of the day but essentially not much changed.

I immediately escaped into a world of denial. I felt I knew my mother better than the doctor and knew what a strong, determined and capable woman she was. I knew my mother would face Alzheimer's with the same strength and courage she'd faced other adversities in her life. I also knew, based on the love and incredibly strong bond between my mother and me, that we would make it to the finish line with this disease without my mother ever forgetting my name or who I was. I was confident my mother would never slip away much beyond the point of mild forgetfulness. If she did, I was equally confident I knew what it meant — and what it would take — to love and care for her. Having watched my mother care for my grandmother, I felt completely prepared and confident for whatever the future would bring our way.

Then, in Thanksgiving, 2004, our lives took another unexpected turn.

♡

Mom had always prepared Thanksgiving dinner by herself, but that year Dad cooked the turkey and I helped Mom prepare the rest of the meal. Mom was agitated which, I believe, was a combination of having Dad and me in "her kitchen" along with the realization that she could no longer prepare meals alone.

Nonetheless, it turned out to be a day filled with great food, conversation, laughter — and one very big surprise.

I was helping my parents clean up after dinner when my dad asked if I'd seen the lumps on Mom's face. Mom turned her face and pointed to the two lumps on her left jawbone. I glanced at Dad.

"We noticed them the other day," he said.

"Do they hurt?" I asked my mother.

"No," she said, feeling them gently with her finger.

The next few weeks passed in a blur of doctor's visits, bloodwork and tests. Just before Christmas, we got the results: non-Hodgkins lymphoma.

Mom looked at the doctor, confused. "It's a form of cancer," the doctor explained and my mother began to cry. Her father had died from stomach cancer and she knew — and feared — what that word meant.

On Christmas Eve, I got an e-mail from a good friend.

> It's 2:00 a.m. I'm here for you. It takes courage to walk this part of the journey, Patti. It takes the love of family and friends. Prayers, memories and laughter... believe it or not, laughter really is the best medicine.
>
> Be well, dear lady. Enjoy this holiday. Nothing needs giving except of the self. Nothing needs to be done or cleaned — it will wait patiently for you. Nothing stands between time's beginning and end except memories worth cherishing. Live them with your whole heart.
>
> Love you,
>
> DJ

The next day, I did exactly what my friend suggested. That Christmas I lived every moment and cherished every memory with my mother, and my family, with my whole heart.

Just after the New Year, Mom began chemotherapy. She was frightened. We all were. She had three treatments a week — each one was three to five hours long. My father and I went along and sat with Mom to keep her company. Mom's oncologist (and the entire staff at the cancer center) were wonderful and made us feel comfortable and confident.

The first few treatments went fairly well but, as the weeks progressed, Mom grew more confused and agitated. When I asked Mom's doctor what was happening, he explained that chemotherapy can impact cognition. Time spent with Mom during her treatments now changed from providing companionship to providing repeated explanations of where we were, why we were there and trying to distract Mom so she wouldn't pull the IV line out of her arm.

After months of chemotherapy, radiation, transfusions, poking and prodding, the doctor proclaimed my mother cancer-free. But those months had left Mom tumbling helplessly down a rabbit hole of confusion. The woman who had entered treatment only mildly confused came out the other end extremely lost and unaware of what she had just gone through.

Mom no longer remembered a time when she didn't wear a wig so long after her own hair grew back, she continued to wear a wig. When her eyelashes, eyebrows and fingernails grew back, she was afraid and thought something was wrong. She had lost a lot of weight, but chemotherapy had changed her taste for many of the foods she always loved so getting her to eat was now a struggle. We may have won the battle with cancer, but we were definitely losing the war with Alzheimer's.

♡

At the time Mom was diagnosed with Alzheimer's, my parents had been married for 60 years. They met in high school. She was a petite, pretty farm girl; he was a tall, handsome football player. After high school graduation, Dad went off to fight in World War II. He was a bellygunner on a B-17, was shot down, taken prisoner and put on a death march. He survived and, after the war ended, he returned home and, once again, crossed paths with my mother. One year later, they were married. My father was a full-time plumber, but spent his nights and weekends building our family a home. Shortly after I was born in 1954, Dad finished the house and we moved in.

My parents were always a team and completely devoted to one another. They worked hard and provided my brother and me with a loving, secure and fun environment to grow up in. We went on family vacations; and on holidays and special occasions, we gathered with our grandparents, aunts, uncles and cousins to celebrate. After my father retired, my parents travelled and enjoyed time with family and a wide circle of friends.

But now, Mom no longer recalled friends' names or faces. She no longer remembered places she and my father had gone or things they'd done together. We watched our father, who had spent a lifetime building memories with his wife, sit in the home he had built for our family and hold onto those memories alone.

♡

One discussion our family never had was who would care for my mother. My brother and I knew the promise our parents had made to one another. Since Dad was in good health, we knew he would be Mom's primary caregiver and my brother and I would support him however and wherever we could. Our family had one goal: to love and care for my mother to the best of our God-given ability.

Without question, my father is the one and only reason we were able to care for my mother at home. Despite the difficulties, heartbreak and exhaustion of caring for my mother, my father rarely (if ever) complained. He was completely and tirelessly devoted to her and her care.

One day, I thanked my father for "doing such a good job with Mom." He turned, looked at me and, in his quiet, gentle way said, "It's not a job, Pat. I love your mother. We married for better or worse and I guess this is the worse part."

I never again called it a "job." My mother was the love of his life and, for my father, caring for her was a labor of love.

♡

I was still working part-time for a local non-profit organization. My boss was very understanding and allowed me to plan my workday around my mother's doctor's appointments and ever-changing needs. My brother, who worked full-time, helped out in the evenings. However, as Mom's Alzheimer's progressed it became obvious that both of my parents needed more help so I quit my job, began to live off my savings, and, together, our family tried to make sense of days filled with the maze and haze of Alzheimer's.

While I was grateful to be able to help my father and care for my mother, I was unprepared for the fear that quickly and completely engulfed me. At times, I was afraid of my mother's behavior and feared I didn't know how to care for her in ways she really needed. I was afraid I wasn't helping my father in ways he really needed, that he would burn out or get sick, and that I would end up losing both of my parents to this disease. I was afraid that, since I'd just given up my job, I would use up my savings and end up in the "poorhouse." I was afraid I'd lose my life — and myself — by caring for my mother. And I was afraid of the disease and that I, like my mother, might one day become one of its unwilling victims.

To help me deal with the onslaught of emotions, I turned to writing. Writing had always helped me make sense of my life and my emotions and it now helped me deal with the fear and confusion that pervaded my life. It also allowed me to vent the frustration and sadness that often welled up inside me.

I wrote on scraps of paper or napkins; I wrote in my journal; and, late at night, I wrote e-mails to friends. E-mail allowed me to stay connected with the outside world to some degree and also became a source of ongoing support and love for me and my family.

From: Patti Kerr
Sent: Tue, 2/15/05 8:03 PM

Greetings Friends and Loved Ones ~

As we continue on this journey with Mom, each day brings a new challenge and a new blessing. Today I went down to help Mom get dressed for her doctor's appointment and she didn't know who I was. Even more astounding, she didn't know my dad. Mom is slipping faster than I ever thought possible. I can't tell you how sad it all makes me.

There's no need to respond to this message. I just

*needed to get it out to the people who understand. I'm so
grateful I have all of you. Thank you for your thoughts,
prayers and e-mails. They mean the world to me — and,
some days, they are the only thing that sustains me during
these challenging times.*

   xo! p.

From: Patti Kerr
Sent: Thur, 5/19/05 3:32 PM

*Dad came around at lunchtime and asked if I wanted
to go to lunch with them. I've learned that's his way of
asking for help and, when I got into their car, I saw how
much he needed help. Mom was having a horrible day.*

*All the way to Dilly's Corner, she kept asking "What's
wrong with me?" I tried to explain that she had shingles
but as soon as I'd finish explaining she'd say, "I don't
understand...what's wrong with me?"*

*She kept asking so finally, halfway through lunch, I
decided to switch tactics and said, "Mom, there's nothing
wrong with you. Why do you think there's something
wrong?" Then she started asking why she had to go to the
doctor...over and over and over again. I finally reached
my limit and said, in an admittedly angry voice, "You
don't have to go to the doctor! We're having lunch and
then going home. Why do you think you have to go to the
doctor?" Mom got really quiet. I felt horrible.*

*On the ride home, I sat in the backseat and looked at
her reflection in the car's mirror. She's gone. Absolutely
gone. Her eyes are completely dead.*

*I felt awful that I'd snapped at her so I tried to make
small talk. Mom stared straight ahead and said, "I don't
know anything. Everybody thinks I'm crazy so I'm not
even gonna talk."*

*Days like these leave me sad and exhausted...and they
seem to be coming closer together.*

*As I sit and write this to all of you, it's obvious to me
now that Mom isn't gone. Just now, as I rewrote our con-*

versation from today, I saw how Mom was still trying to ask appropriate questions and understand what is happening to her. The problem wasn't her; it was <u>me</u>. The problem was that I didn't know how to give her the answers in a way she could understand.

So I'm sad that, more and more often, I no longer know how to communicate with my mother. I believe if I can figure out that one very important puzzle piece it could make a huge difference in our daily life — if only for a while.

xo! p.

My mother loved music. Polkas, country western, rock and roll, you name it — Mom loved it. I have vivid memories of my mother cleaning house on Saturday mornings, music blasting as she danced with the vacuum cleaner.

After Alzheimer's, music remained a constant source of joy in my mother's life and, on her most difficult days, music was the one thing that, more often than not, would calm her down. It also created special moments — and memories.

For years, my parents and many of their friends had gone on Saturday night to a local radio station's live country music show. Now, to allow Dad time to rest (or watch his beloved New York Yankees), I began taking Mom on Saturday nights. Many of my parents' friends still went to the show, but Mom no longer recognized them. They would smile and wave at her. She would smile and wave back, but had no idea who they were.

One Saturday in August 2006, I invited a friend who was visiting from out-of-town to join Mom and me. He'd never met my mother before, but we all had a wonderful time together. Afterwards, he sent me this e-mail:

Your Mama is a hoot! I wish I'd had the chance to get to know her before all of this, but I'm so grateful I got to meet her now. It feels like on some level she knows things aren't quite right and that some of the things she does are a way of coping with it. But then she drifts back to the place that none of us can know...and only wonder about. — G

Even though Mom began to drift more and more to that place my friend talked about, music remained a constant and consistent way to reach and communicate with her. And, for my father, it created precious moments with his wife.

One afternoon, as I approached my parents' front door, I heard music playing. I quietly opened the door and tiptoed down the hall. Peeking around the corner, I saw my parents dancing in the other room.

They were dancing like I'd seen them do thousands of times in my life. But this time it was different. The way my father gently held my mother as they danced and the way she looked up at him, smiling, was special. Even the words to the song my father was singing to my mother — Eddie Arnold's "Make The World Go Away" — held special significance. *"Make the world go away and get it all off my shoulders...say the things you used to say and make the world go away..."*

I stood out of sight. They hadn't heard me come in and didn't know I was there. They were completely lost in the moment — and each other. I didn't want to interrupt them, so I snapped a quick photo with my cell phone and quietly left. Now, when I look at that picture, I don't see Alzheimer's. I see two people in love.

Despite all Mom had forgotten, she still remembered where I lived and, since we only lived a few houses apart, Mom walked back and forth between my house and theirs all day long.

No matter how much time I spent at their house, as soon as I left, Mom would be at my front door. She'd knock quietly and when I came to the door, she'd smile as if she hadn't seen me for months. We'd sit on the couch and talk. She'd tell me what a nice house I had, as if she'd never seen it before. Sometimes, we'd watch family movies.

My mother no longer recognized herself or anyone else in the movies. She didn't realize the people in the movie were her family and people she'd known for years. When she saw my dad, my brother, my sons or me in the movies, she'd ask me who "those people" were. I'd just smile, hug my mother and tell her they were all people who loved her.

One afternoon, the doorbell rang. My son Sean answered the door. It was our mailman, Mike.

"I just saw your grandmother up on Broad Street," Mike said. He told Sean he'd said hello but she seemed confused and lost so he hopped into his mail truck and came to our house to tell us.

Sean ran to find his grandmother. Luckily, she had only gone a few blocks. Approaching her very calmly, he said, "Hi, Grandma." She looked at him, smiled, and said, "My boy." He put his arm around her and, together, they slowly walked back home.

I believe my mother had, like she did every day, walked up the street to visit me but, for the first time, she hadn't recognized my house and kept on walking.

After that, we kept an even closer watch on Mom and made sure she never left the house alone. A few months later, she gave us another scare.

Mom entered a very difficult phase where, as we approached dinnertime, she would begin to get very agitated. It was difficult — and sometimes impossible — to calm her down. Many nights, instead of sleeping, Mom wandered around the house, disoriented and agitated. My father followed behind her to make sure she was safe. Sometimes she — and my father — went days without sleeping. My father was completely exhausted so, during the day, when Mom was calmer, I would bring her to my house and give Dad a chance to sleep.

At the time, I didn't know enough about Alzheimer's to know what to do or even that the behavior had a name: sundowning. All I knew was my grandmother had gone through it and I remembered what it had done to my mother. It had completely worn her out — and had ultimately brought about the family's decision to place my grandmother in a nursing home.

One morning when I arrived at my parents' house, Mom was agitated. I knew taking her to my house would only escalate the situation so my father and I turned to music to try and calm her down. Many polka records later, Mom relaxed and, soon after, fell into a deep sleep. My father said he, too, was going to try and get some sleep so I tiptoed out and went home.

An hour later, my phone rang. "Is your mother there?" my dad asked.

"No."

"She's gone. I can't find her," he said. I could hear the fear in his voice.

"I'm on my way," I said hanging up the phone. As I ran down the street, I called out for my mother. When I got to my parents' house, Dad was panicked.

"I didn't even hear her leave," he said. "I woke up and she was gone."

As we walked outside to begin searching the neighborhood, we looked down the street and saw a police car, a young couple — and my mother.

Dad and I walked down the street and, when Mom saw us, she smiled and said, "Here they are," as if nothing had happened.

"Hi, Mom. You okay?"

"Yeah, why?"

"Just asking. Where were you going?"

"Nowhere. What do you mean?"

My father began slowly walking my mother home while I remained behind to find out what had happened. The young couple said they had seen my mother walking down the street towards the highway and grew concerned because she seemed confused and disoriented. As they approached her their suspicions were confirmed and they called 911. They stayed and talked with my mom until the police officer and my father and I arrived. I answered the officer's questions and then ran to catch up to my parents.

As I walked besides my mother, I asked her where she'd been going. She laughed and said she was looking for me. My father and I glanced at each other, knowing that, once again, Mom had changed the rules and the stakes were getting higher.

For me, along with the moments of frustration and exhaustion that accompanied caring for Mom (and worrying about Dad) were moments of pure joy. Joy in little things: giving Mom a manicure, going for walks, holding her hand, dancing the polka with her, watching her eyes light up when my sons entered the room, and listening to her laugh and smile at my father. Moments spent doing what, before Alzheimer's, had been seemingly inconsequential things took on special — and monumental — meaning.

In the evening, after dinner, my brother, my father, my mother and I would sit on their back deck and talk. Night after night, Mom told us the story of how she and her girlfriends used to stare at my dad in high school. No matter how many times she told the story, my dad would always smile and blush.

I didn't realize how much I loved hearing that story, or how much I liked seeing my father smile and blush, until Mom stopped telling it. When we never heard the story again, I realized just how sacred those evenings on the back deck were.

I realized, through this journey with my mother, how much time, effort and needless worry is spent on things people assume are more important: a job or career, money, big houses, fancy cars. Yet none of that could (or would) have ever changed the path we were on with my Mom.

In the end, none of that mattered. What mattered was that we took the time to sit on the deck every night and talk and listen to Mom tell her story.

♡

My mother had always been a loving, caring, generous wife, mother and grandmother. She had also been a "take charge" kind of woman which, at times, made her seem harsh and controlling. After Alzheimer's, Mom lost the need (or ability) to take charge and be in control. Instead, she gained a whole new level of softness and tenderness. She became even more loving and grateful — and she expressed it freely and constantly. She thanked everyone repeatedly for everything and told us over and over how much she loved us. She became even more playful and danced regardless of who was watching.

I've often wondered if, as Alzheimer's progressed, it had dissolved my mother's defense mechanisms thereby allowing us to see her — her true essence and who she truly was — absent of any fear or concern. I used to think how wonderful it would be if we all were able to operate without fear, allow our pure essence to shine, and dance regardless of who was watching.

On Halloween 2006, my life began to spin out of control — only this time it had nothing to do with my mother.

My husband, who had recently gone for a check-up, was diagnosed with a potentially life-threatening illness. He didn't want anyone other than me to know. So now, in addition to being a caregiver for my mother, I became his sole confidant and source of support.

Since I held my husband's secret, my e-mails from that time only tell half the story.

From: Patti Kerr
Sent: Wed., 12/13/06 1:06 AM

My dear friends and family ~

I'm sorry I've been difficult to reach lately. I'm on a wild ride right now. There's a lot coming at me from all angles and I'm trying as hard as I can to hang on. I thought the roller coaster ride was intense before but I've now tightened my seat belt even more.

I'm covered in a rash from head to toe. I could say I don't know what it's from but I think I do — it's the stress. My doctor said to take Benadryl to relieve the itching. I had no idea Benadryl makes you tired so I took one while I was still at Mom and Dad's and, soon after, started getting woozy. I fell asleep in my old bedroom at their house and slept for five hours. Right before I fell asleep, Mom blew her nose and started shoving the tissue in her mouth to eat it. Gratefully, Dad was with her or I don't know what I would have found when I woke up.

I'll be in touch when time/energy/desire coincide. Wishing all of you a holiday filled with love, laughter and magical moments.

xo! p.

Two weeks later, and two days after Christmas, I sent a follow-up e-mail:

From: Patti Kerr
Sent: Wed., 12/27/06 1:06 AM

Happy belated holidays. I'm sorry this is late but, once again, Mom isn't sleeping at night. I remember when my grandmother went through this and the family had to take turns staying with her so they could all get enough sleep. My dad is being stoic and brave, but today he dozed off and woke up to the sound of the doorbell. Mom had wandered out and the neighbor saw her walking around aimlessly, without a coat, in the cold and wind.

I also find it's difficult to write to all of you right now because it's almost like I can't relate to the real world anymore. The outside world is so far removed from what I'm experiencing, and have been experiencing for so long, that it's tough for me to hear about how normal people live. In all honesty, it also makes me jealous. Sometimes I wonder what it would feel like to have a life — my life — back again. And there's no end in sight.

I'm exhausted...burned out...spent. I think I'm going to go make tea and crawl into bed. May the New Year bring all of us an abundance of health, joy and laughter.

xo! p.

Since I wasn't able to tell my father what was happening with my husband, I had to constantly find new excuses for not being there to help him with my mother. I also felt caught between the proverbial "rock and a hard place" and carried guilt with me no matter where I went or what I did. If I was helping my husband, I felt guilty my father didn't have any help. If I was helping my father, I felt guilty my husband was alone.

I remember people telling me how strong I was or how "God only gives you what you can handle." When people told me that, I wanted to say: "Well, then, it looks like I need to send God a note and let him know he's got me confused with someone else because I'm really *not* that strong."

♡

By the spring of 2007, my husband was given a clean bill of health. However, since I'd been ignoring my own health, I had developed my own problems and was scheduled for surgery. The surgeon said I'd be unable to help with Mom's care for a minimum of four weeks since caring for Mom now included helping her with toileting and, in doing that, I ran an increased risk of getting an infection after surgery.

Together, Dad and I had our hands full with my mother. We were struggling to find anything Mom would eat. She had become completely resistant to my attempts to wash her hair or bathe her. She was hallucinating — seeing people lurking in corners and convinced the people on the TV were really inside their house. Mom grew increasingly agitated and confused as the line between fantasy and reality continued to fade.

With my surgery scheduled, I felt additional pressure to get things under control. I knew Dad couldn't handle it on his own so I talked to him about getting additional help during those four weeks. Unconvinced he needed help, Dad reluctantly agreed to consider it. I knew he needed the help — I also knew I was coming undone as the entry from my journal at that time clearly shows.

June 28, 2007

> *I'm falling apart and, even though he won't admit it, Dad is, too. He's visibly agitated and frustrated.*
>
> *I arranged for a home health aide to come in and help while I'm recuperating from surgery but I think Dad's already decided it won't work. I pray I'm wrong because if this doesn't work, I don't know what to do.*
>
> *Yesterday, when I told him the home health aide was coming at 12:30 to meet him and Mom, he said, "You'll be here, right?" I reminded Dad I had to leave at 1:00 to go for my pre-op tests and he just shook his head in disgust — as if I was choosing the tests over helping him care for Mom. Trust me, I'd prefer not to have surgery this summer but that's the harsh reality.*
>
> *Sometimes I feel like I just can't do it anymore. I've*

come to the realization that I'm not the person my father is. He made the commitment to Mom "for better or worse" but I didn't and sometimes all I want is to get a piece of my life back. At this point, I can't make any plans or do anything because I never know what the day will hold.

It's also frustrating because I still have no idea how to communicate with Dad. Whenever I leave their house, I always tell him to let me know if he or Mom needs something. He never calls but yet, when I go down there he's all pissed off because he needed to go to the store and "there's no way I can get out of the house." No matter how many times I tell him he should have called, he doesn't and he won't.

My doctor wants to up my daily dose of Zoloft from 75 mg. a day (the same drug and dosage they have Mom on for depression) to 200 mg. a day. I don't want to do that. Honestly, I look forward to the day when I won't be on anti-depressants anymore.

I started seeing my therapist again. She is wonderful and has a calming, hopeful effect on me. I was supposed to meet with her today before I went for my pre-op tests but had to cancel because the home health aide was starting and Dad wanted me to "be there to get her going." Anyway, my therapist told me I'm severely depressed and overwhelmed which I already knew. I spend more and more time in bed...I don't want to get up...but, in the middle of the night, I lie there for hours and mull the whole situation over and over in my head. I don't know how to extract myself — even just a little — to get "me" back. I don't know where the line is between being a "good daughter" and having a life.

These are the thoughts rolling around in my head these days. When I'm down there, I just want to get the hell out. It's so depressing and wears me out. When I'm not there, I feel guilty that I'm not there and that Dad is handling it all by himself. So what do I do?!?! Where do I go from here?!?!?

I'm falling apart, piece by piece...and the pace is pick-
ing up. God help me.
  xo! p.

The home health aide started the day I went for surgery. On her second day, my father fired her, saying he could care for my mother on his own. Two weeks after my surgery, despite my doctor's orders and stern warnings, I returned to help my dad care for my mother.

On September 19, 2007, we celebrated my mother's 82nd birthday. Since she loved chocolate, and since she was no longer able to use utensils, I decided to make her favorite chocolate cupcakes. We sang "Happy Birthday" as Mom laughed and clapped along.

The next day, Mom tripped and cut her chin. When she tried to get up off the floor, she grabbed at her hip and winced in pain, unable to tell us what was wrong or what she felt. My father and I called 911.

An ambulance took Mom to the hospital where she got stitches in her chin and X-rays of her hip. The X-ray showed a minor fracture in her pelvis and the hospital said they were going to keep Mom overnight for observation. My father and I were afraid being away from home would cause Mom additional stress but the hospital assured us she would be fine. We checked on her by phone over the next several hours and, after being repeatedly assured she'd been sedated for the pain and was sleeping soundly, we finally stopped calling and went to bed.

The next morning, the hospital informed us Mom was being transferred to a nearby rehab facility for physical therapy. A week later, the rehab facility told us physical therapy wasn't possible due to her advanced Alzheimer's and suggested she be transferred to their Alzheimer's wing.

While I was concerned for my mother, I was more concerned for my father. He couldn't accept that Mom's fall had been an unavoidable accident and continued to blame himself. Every time we visited my mother, my father left more sullen and somber than the time before. He desperately wanted to bring Mom home.

The facility, on the other hand, told me they believed Mom

was too advanced for us to care for her at home and that, unless we got additional help at home, they would fight our request to release Mom back to our care.

♡

Dad hung on the best he could. I, on the other hand, began to spiral downward along with Mom. I had run out of steam and decided the only solution was to run away from my life.

October 24, 2007

To the men in my life,
    I have run away. It's not important you know where I've gone but it is important you know why.
    I'm burned out...fried...exhausted. If I don't do this, I honestly feel I will have a breakdown and that is simply not an option for me...

This is a portion of the letter I left for my father, brother, sons and husband before hopping in my car and driving away. I didn't know where I was going. I only knew I was losing my grip.

An hour later, I stumbled upon a beautiful resort and spa. I checked in and, for the next three days, I slept, got massages, took walks, wrote, sat in silence and thought. At the end of the three days, I checked out and drove home. My first stop was to visit my mother. I sat with her for hours and it was one of the most relaxed visits I'd had with her in a long time. I was refreshed, renewed and reenergized.

During those three days, I learned that none of the men in my life were responsible for what I'd been feeling. For years, I had been too proud to ask for help and had ignored all signs of burnout. I wanted to be, and often thought I was, Superwoman. But, in Alzheimer's, I'd met an adversary that was taking away the best parts of me, little by little and piece by piece — and, to a large degree, I had stood by and willingly allowed it to happen.

During those three days, and after years of caring for my mother, I had finally learned the **#1 Rule of Caregiving: Take care of yourself first.** Unfortunately, although I didn't know it at the time, I learned the lesson very late in the game. My mother only had a few months to live.

Several months before my mother's fall, I had attended my first meeting of our local Alzheimer's caregivers support group. At that meeting, a woman had told the group about a wonderful caregiver who was available. I hadn't paid attention since, at that time, we didn't need anyone. However, our situation was now very different so I got the caregiver's number and made arrangements for my father and me to meet her.

Bernice walked into my father's house and we both immediately liked her. However, my father and I knew the most important connection needed to happen between Bernice and my mom so we all got into the car and drove over to the facility.

Mom hadn't walked since the day of the accident so we weren't surprised to find her alone in her room, strapped into a wheelchair.

As we walked towards my mother, she looked up at my father and me — and then at Bernice. She held her hands up, Bernice bent down, and my mother took Bernice's face in her hands and smiled. I knew the interview was over and that Mom had just found the final member of her caregiving team.

♡

The facility brought hospice on board due to the advancement of Mom's Alzheimer's so, when we got home from our visit, I called hospice and told them we wanted to bring Mom home. Together, we put a plan in place. Within 48 hours, due to the hard work and sheer determination of our family — and the help of hospice — the house was ready for Mom's homecoming. At long last, I saw the spark return to my father's eyes. His wife was coming home.

On the morning we arrived to bring Mom home, we were warned by the facility that Mom had adjusted so well to being there that she would probably go through a difficult transition period. We decided to take our chances.

The medical transport van arrived and when they wheeled Mom in she was completely calm and unaffected. When we arrived home, they opened the door to the van and Mom sat in her wheelchair, smiling. We brought her into the house, she looked around, smiled, and dozed off for a nap. We never had one second of difficulty with her. She slept, ate, and was calm. Even though she couldn't say it, my mother knew she was home.

Equally important, my father, once again, was doing what he wanted to do more than anything in the world: he was caring for his wife in their home just as he'd always promised he would.

Hospice was now our sacred, valued partner in caring for Mom. They taught us how to keep Mom comfortable and content. They told us to keep the room warm and the lights lowered. They explained that hearing was the last sense to leave a person and, knowing how much my mother loved music, we kept music quietly playing in the room for her. We also told her repeatedly how much we loved her.

As the weeks passed, Mom began to eat less and sleep more. Our natural instincts were to try to find something she would eat but hospice gently explained her lack of appetite and increased sleeping were normal since Mom was nearing the end of her journey.

At first, we didn't believe them and kept trying to find something — anything — she would eat. We wanted to prove them wrong, to prove this wasn't the end — but just a detour — on our journey with her through Alzheimer's. But as the weeks passed, it became obvious they were right.

After Thanksgiving dinner, knowing how much my mother loved Christmas, we put up my parents' Christmas tree in the living room. We also decorated Mom's room and played Christmas carols for her. We wanted, in whatever way possible, to celebrate Christmas with her one last time. And then, one by one, we went in to say our final goodbyes.

Every second of every day, I found myself holding my breath, wondering if today would be the day. Yet every day, Mom clung to life — and I clung to her.

On December 3rd, after spending the morning with Mom, and seeing she was calm and relaxed, my father and I decided to go to the grocery store to get a few things we needed. It was the first time we'd left my mother's side in weeks. We kissed her and told her we'd be right back. Her eyes remained closed and she remained calm.

I glanced at my watch when we left the grocery store. It was 12:30, lunchtime. We called home and Bernice assured us Mom was fine. We told her we were going to pick up lunch and would be right home.

We arrived home approximately 15 minutes later. Typically, the first thing I would do was go into Mom's room to see her and make sure she was alright. I don't know why, this time, I didn't. Instead, I sat down to have lunch with my dad and Bernice, but a few minutes later, something told me to stop and go check on Mom. I excused myself and got up from the table. When I walked into her room, I knew. Mom was gone.

As we sat and quietly ate lunch, Mom had taken advantage of those few minutes alone to make her quiet exit from this world.

Their Journey with Alzheimer's

Alzheimer's doesn't discriminate. It strikes our neighbors, co-workers and the man we pass on the street as well as Presidents, Prime Ministers, authors, college professors, and celebrities. Whoever and whatever we are — and whatever awards, accolades, social status or riches we've achieved — no longer matter. Since there is no typical or predicable path the disease follows, everyone's journey with — and story about — Alzheimer's is different.

When I began writing this book, I hoped our family's experience could help another individual or family who might one day walk in our footsteps. However, we were just one voice and one experience with Alzheimer's. I knew for the book to be truly helpful to others, it needed the stories, voices and experiences of others who had loved and cared for a parent with Alzheimer's.

Gratefully, there were many sons, daughters and grandchildren who were willing to share their experience, wisdom and insight. In this chapter, and every chapter that follows, you will meet them and hear about their journey with their parent and Alzheimer's. By including a variety of caregivers' stories and voices, I hope you will find an individual (or several) who will resonate with you and assist you on your journey.

Note: Stories and advice from caregivers throughout the book are arranged in alphabetical order by the caregiver's first name for quick and easy future reference.

ALLYSON'S JOURNEY: For Me, It's A Gift

Before our family knew Dad had dementia, we felt he should be living in a more social environment. Mom died several years earlier and Dad was living alone in a development where most of his neighbors worked all day. We all thought a move would give him opportunities to do things with people his own age. We found an active adult community which was still being built and signed a contract for a two-story townhouse. We were planning ahead. Our thought was, if Dad's health declined, we could hire someone to live with him in the upstairs bedroom.

After we signed the contract, we began to see that Dad was getting very confused, losing all concept of time, and was having trouble with his finances. One time, when I visited, I noticed there were teabags burned in the bottom of a frying pan. When I asked him about it, he said his microwave was broken and he was trying to make himself a cup of tea.

Dad's physician suggested I take him to a neurologist to be tested. Originally, he was diagnosed with mild cognitive impairment but, within a year, the diagnosis was changed to Alzheimer's. I believe Dad is currently in the middle stages of Alzheimer's.

I'd been working for the same company for almost 20 years. I continued to work after Dad's diagnosis, but eventually, as Dad's problems became too difficult to manage long-distance, I took a family leave.

One of the benefits from my employment was a geriatric assessment of a parent. At Dad's assessment, they recommended he be placed in an assisted living facility. I did an in-depth evaluation of the ones in our area and took Dad to see one I thought he might like. When we arrived, there were several people sleeping in the lobby. Dad hated it and absolutely refused to go.

I have two brothers and a sister and some of them have children or are dealing with their own personal health issues. Since my husband and I don't have any children and are fortunate to have the room and financial resources to care for him, I was the obvious choice to be Dad's caregiver. I decided to take an early retirement so I could care for Dad. When Dad asked about my job, I told him I'd taken a leave to see whether or not I wanted to retire.

The ultimate goal was to have Dad move in with us so I began to take gradual steps in that direction. I'd stay at his house, or he'd stay with us, and, over time, he got very used to being with me. I also began to do all the driving so he got out of the habit of driving.

I then told Dad if we waited until his townhouse was ready before selling his house we could end up with two houses to maintain. He agreed, so we got his house ready and, thankfully, it sold quickly.

Since his new townhouse still wasn't going to be ready for another six months, Dad moved in with us. Once he was settled, we began talking about how far away his new townhouse was from our house. I told him we'd love to have him move in with us and that he could help me with my garden. By that point, I think Dad realized he was declining and was relieved to have a way to maintain his pride and also feel he would be a big help to us if he stayed here.

I'm very fortunate to have a husband who is supportive and helps wherever and whenever he can. This hasn't always been easy on him. There have been a lot of changes since Dad moved in. We can't go out to dinner alone or on vacation. On the rare occasion we do go away, my brothers or sister come and stay at the house so Dad's routine isn't disrupted. But, since they have their own medical issues and children, they can only stay for short periods of time.

About a year ago, Dad started getting angry when my husband was around and kept threatening to leave. Last Memorial Day, he did.

We'd been at the town parade and, when we got home, my husband went to take a nap. Dad said he was going to lie down, too. I was working on the computer but kept checking on Dad every hour. The first two times I checked on him, he was sound asleep. The third time, he was gone. He'd left a note on a napkin saying he was going for a walk. I hopped in the car and finally found him about five miles away walking along the highway.

I think Dad wandered back to the town park because there was a picnic and lots of children. He loved children. I think on his way back home he missed the turn for our road and just kept walking.

I immediately had alarms installed on the doors and in the driveway to alert us if Dad ever decides to leave the house unaccompanied again.

I also made fliers on my computer with Dad's picture and vital information (height, weight, age, that he has Alzheimer's, is physically fit and can walk very quickly) along with contact information for our family. I gave copies of the flier to family, friends and neighbors and the local police. I'm considering registering Dad in the Safe Return program that's available in our county but I don't know if he'll wear the ID bracelet which is a critical part of the program.

After the wandering incident, I had another geriatric assessment done. This time, they recommended Dad go to a local adult day program. Initially, it was very difficult for him to adjust, but now he loves it and thinks he works there.

It's also been a huge help to me because it allows me time to myself each day. It's impossible for me to watch Dad all day, every day, so this has made it possible for me to keep him at home.

I had to make changes in our home to keep Dad safe. Since he still dresses and bathes himself, I simplified his bathroom and removed anything that could confuse him or be a potential danger — cleaners, medication, excess decorations and rugs. I also found light strips in the Vermont Country Store catalog which I put on the bathroom tile and floor. That, along with nightlights, helps direct Dad if he gets up during the night to use the bathroom.

I had to simplify and remove any clutter throughout the rest of the house, especially in his room. However, I wanted Dad's room to feel homey, so I put family photos and other things that are important to him in his room. I got a dry-erase board and every day Dad and I write the day of the week, the weather, and what activities he'll be doing that day on the board. Every evening, before bed, we sit together and talk about what he'll be doing the next day. I bought him a clock with a large digital display which shows the day of the week, the date and the time. I'm trying to keep him alert and aware for as long as possible.

Every night, I lay out his clothes for the next day. Dad doesn't always put those clothes on, and some of his outfits are quite interesting, but I don't say anything. It really doesn't matter.

I know it's important to find small tasks Dad can complete successfully and with pride so, since he always loved gardening, I look for things he can do in the garden. I work alongside him or monitor him constantly, even if he's outside for only a short period of time.

My biggest fear for the future is that there might come a time when I can no longer care for my father. I know there is a possibility we might one day have to place him in a residential facility and, in fact, I have his name on two waiting lists already. That's when my brothers and sister will have to step in because taking him to a facility will just be too painful for me.

Attitude is everything. I never criticize Dad. If he puts something where it doesn't belong I don't correct him. I just fix it later. I make changes gradually. What's worked for me is to stay calm and consistent and to praise him constantly. We also tell lots of jokes.

Dad is a sweetheart. He's an absolute delight and is fine in almost every social situation. He genuinely enjoys being around people, and they enjoy him. I love seeing him enjoy life and time with his family.

I'm not saying everybody should do what I did. But, for me, it's been a gift to spend time with him while he is still aware, delightful and appreciative. I feel I'm giving back for all the years my parents cared for all of us.

♡

AMI'S JOURNEY: An Only Child In Charge of Mom's Care

My mother was a free spirit. She was a creative, unconventional and exuberant soul. She was quirky, eccentric and chronically happy. She was a hoot! My mother never complained but chose instead to find beauty everywhere she looked.

Before Alzheimer's, my mother:

- brought near-dead orchid plants home from local nurseries and nursed them back to health.

- made her own clothes, mostly in bright, garish colors.

- cut her own hair (badly).

- cursed like a sailor.

- bought skylights and coffin liners and made them into ponds for her yard.

- talked to strangers all the time.

- exaggerated constantly.

- never followed directions.

- was fearless.

- did what she wanted when she wanted to do it.

- went to clown college when she was in her 70s to entertain old people.

Mom was my best friend and, even though we visited each other often, I didn't have a clue anything was wrong until she complained of not being able to read. I went with her to the doctor and, first, she couldn't remember where the office was; and then, when we finally got there, I discovered she hadn't been taking some of her medication.

The doctor suggested that, instead of reading, my mother try listening to books on tape but Mom couldn't figure out how to work the tape recorder. We switched doctors and Mom began undergoing tests to determine what was wrong. We also began looking back and realized there had been other signs: problems while driving, seeing colors that weren't there, lapses in logic, and notes sprouting from every surface in her home.

Mom was diagnosed with Alzheimer's in 2001. My father had passed away in 1984 at the age of 60. I'm an only child. I've heard, from talking with other families who had a loved one with Alzheimer's, being an only child was a blessing because I was in charge of Mom's care. The bad thing about it was *I was in charge of Mom's care!*

When Mom was diagnosed, I lived about 60 miles away and made weekly, then twice-a-week, visits to help her. My husband, my mother and I also designed and built an addition to our home with the idea that, when she grew tired of living by herself, she would move in with us. However, when the addition was done, Mom refused to move. I would badger her to move in; she would tell me to bug off.

She finally moved in right after 9/11 and lived with us for over four years. I don't know what actually made her decide to move in with us — and I never asked. I was just grateful she did.

My husband and daughter helped care for Mom and, since I have a home-based business, several employees also pitched in.

I always thought my "line in the sand" for moving Mom out of our home and into a care facility would be when she became incontinent. That was mainly because I knew when I had to leave our home for business I wouldn't be able to ask my husband to change my mother's diaper.

As it turned out, the "line in the sand" came way before that when Mom tried to "go home," scantily-clad, and wandered out of the house at 3:00 AM in 20 degree weather. Gratefully, I noticed the front door was open.

Before this incident, we never left Mom alone and rarely went out by ourselves. Since I work out of our home, I could either work or take care of Mom — not both — so we hired people to watch Mom during the day. We had people in our house all day long and now, with Mom's attempted escape, it would mean we'd have people in the house at night, too, since she now needed 24-hour care.

We moved Mom into an assisted living facility that was, literally, 90 seconds from our house. She lived there for about three years before being moved to hospice.

Around the time my mother moved into the assisted living, I founded the Alzheimer's Art Quilt Initiative. Two years later, in 2008, it became a national nonprofit charity with supporters throughout the United States. We are a volunteer grassroots effort whose mission is to raise awareness and fund research for Alzheimer's through art.

♡

ANN'S JOURNEY: Blessed To Have Her

My husband, Tom, and I have been married for over 35 years and have three daughters and one grandchild.

Tom and I first suspected something was wrong when Mom began leaving key ingredients out of recipes, was asking the same questions over and over, and couldn't remember the day or date. As time passed, it got worse.

In September 2005, my husband, Mom and I went to Nebraska for my 35th class reunion. On the airplane, Mom was extremely confused and kept asking why we were there and why the airplane wasn't moving. She was moody and somewhat paranoid on the trip and sometimes lapsed into a semi-sleep state and began talking to herself.

The night after we arrived home from our trip, Mom had an incident at the senior apartment complex where she lived. Her apartment was on the second floor, but Mom was on the first floor, in her nightgown, completely lost and disoriented. Management warned us if Mom was no longer cognizant of her surroundings, she couldn't live there any longer.

Several months later, when Mom was outside her apartment refusing to go back in because there were "men in her apartment," we were asked to find another place for her to live.

Mom moved into an assisted living apartment complex and, on the advice of her general practitioner, I took Mom to a neurologist who told us she had Alzheimer's and put her on Aricept.

Mom never accepted the diagnosis. She said she would fight it by exercising and keeping her mind active. She got subscriptions to several Alzheimer's newsletters, researched as much as she could, and worked really hard at staying alert. She read, did crossword puzzles every day, and watched the news to keep up on current events.

Despite all she was doing, the one thing she wouldn't do was talk about it. We never talked about her diagnosis or Alzheimer's. Mom felt if she didn't talk about something, it didn't exist. She'd done that her whole life and it certainly wasn't any different now.

When I tried to bring it up for discussion, she'd change the subject. She was good at denial.

My own feelings ran from denial to anger to fear. Mom was very loving, incredibly smart, well-spoken and opinionated and I didn't want to watch her be reduced to anything less. I didn't want her mind and memories taken away.

I was also very upset because Mom had told me numerous times she could handle anything except losing her mind. After her diagnosis, she told me (on more than one occasion) that "the worse thing in the world would be to lose my mind" and that she "didn't want to live that way."

I was also afraid I might inherit the disease.

For a while, I didn't think Mom was that bad. Her Alzheimer's seemed to plateau which made it easier for me to believe she didn't have the disease. Even though I verbalized that she had it, in the deepest part of me I didn't want to believe it. It was the only way I could cope.

My brother spoke with Mom regularly but he didn't think she was "all that bad." He didn't realize Mom was making notes to keep things straight and so she wouldn't repeat anything during their conversations. When I told him, we began to talk about what we would do as the disease progressed. However, since he lived halfway across the country, it was difficult for him to actually be in on any of the decisions.

Gratefully, my husband and three grown daughters helped. My mother always loved my husband like a son and my daughters were very close to their grandmother so they were excellent sounding boards.

My father had died in January 2003 and that had been awful for Mom. Now, years later and only four months after my mother was diagnosed with Alzheimer's, my brother was diagnosed with cancer. He died five months later and, after his death, Mom really started to decline. She couldn't accept my brother's death and constantly said she wished it had been her and that "no parent should outlive a child." Honestly, I believe from that point on, Mom just wanted to die.

In September 2007, two years after her diagnosis, Mom stopped going to church. She was embarrassed she could no longer remember people's names, had begun speaking out during times of silence, and was having trouble determining what behavior was appropriate.

Mom's medication was causing diarrhea and vomiting and she began having increased episodes of incontinence. Since she felt sick most of the time, she wasn't eating very much. A decision was made to take her off Aricept — and then the freefall really began.

Mom was still able to dress herself and go down to eat meals with the others who lived at the complex. Then, in late November, she was constantly looking for my father and brother (both deceased) or me. She would call me on the phone and tell me she was lost when, in fact, she was inside her apartment.

Then Mom began needing more assistance with her daily life. The staff really liked her and would go up to Mom's apartment to remind her to come down for meals or help her get dressed. I'm not sure if they were supposed to do those things but I'm grateful they did.

At the end of December, Mom fell and cracked her pelvis. Since she could no longer stay in assisted living, while she was recovering, one of my daughters and her friends helped me move Mom's belongings from the assisted living to the nursing home next door. That move was more difficult than I thought it would be.

Since I didn't want Mom to stay in the nursing home, I found a residential home for Alzheimer's patients. It wasn't covered by insurance, but they were wonderful, and since they only housed six patients, I knew Mom would get very personalized care. Since it was less than a mile from our home, I visited every day — and watched Mom's quick descent.

Some days, she was almost lucid and realized "something wasn't right." She would ask me if she was losing her mind. My heavens, that was difficult.

I was lucky. She knew who I was up until two days before she died. She told me she loved me and was blessed to have a daughter like me. I know I was blessed to have a mom like her.

♡

CHARLIE'S JOURNEY:
Great Way To Pay Him Back

In June 2003, when my father was 86, he was diagnosed with Lewy body dementia, which has some of the same symptoms and pattern of decline as Alzheimer's. At the time, I was living in Illinois and my father was living outside Boston with his second wife, Anne.

The reason for his diagnosis was twofold. First, it was based on discussions my father and I had over a nine month period where he kept telling me he was having increased difficulty with his handwriting. He said it felt like the pen was jumping in the middle of a sentence for no reason. He stopped driving because he felt his reactions weren't what they used to be. He was also having difficulty balancing his checkbook, which was completely out of character since he had always been brilliant with any kind of math or calculations. The only other person he shared these symptoms with was his primary care physician who told him it was simply that he was "getting old."

The second reason came out of the blue. In the spring of 2003, I received a phone call from my stepmother at 1:00 AM telling me I should fly to Boston as soon as possible to see my father because he "didn't have long to live and was fading fast." My stepmother had been diagnosed with cancer several months before, and my father had been going with her to her oncology appointments. At one of the appointments, her oncologist told her that, based on his observations, he believed my father had some form of dementia, probably Alzheimer's. Unfortunately, the doctor also told my stepmother it was incurable and that he felt my father would "most likely die in a few months." Gratefully, my stepmother and the doctor had decided not to tell my father about the "diagnosis" because they wanted him to "die with dignity." I immediately got on a plane to Boston.

My wife works at a nursing home and got the name of a geriatric specialist in Boston. My father and I spent three hours with the specialist. She talked to my father, gave him standard memory tests, checked him physically and reviewed his gait and balance.

At the end of the appointment, she said the results pointed to Lewy body dementia and then explained the disease to us.

I immediately fired my father's primary care physician and trusted my father's care to this new doctor. We also honored my father's request to know everything that was going on with him and did so until he passed away. I believe it gave him a sense of control.

I then flew back to Illinois but returned regularly for doctor visits. We kept that routine up for about four months. My step-mother was still undergoing treatment for cancer and, despite help from her family, she was having increased difficulty caring for my dad. After my father came to stay with us for a short visit, I decided it was best if he moved to Illinois and lived with my wife and me and, in the interim, my stepmother passed away.

I was very lucky to have a spouse who "got it" and took my father into our home without hesitation and treated him like a king.

We got Dad into an adult day program a couple of times a week and got help on the days he was home so my wife and I could continue to work. After a few months, I was laid off so I began caring for my father full-time.

Eight months later, a room opened in the dementia care facility where my wife worked so we moved my father onto a floor that had 24-hour nurses and staff. Since it was only six blocks from our home, I visited every day and sometimes several times a day.

Having the nursing home within a ten minute walk of my house allowed me to check in on my father at a moment's notice. Because I was there so often, I was involved in all of Dad's caregiving decisions. I also discussed any huge decisions with my sister.

I was very lucky Dad planned his finances as well as he did because it meant I didn't have to return to work but could focus on taking care of him. It meant I was able to monitor his care and quality of life on a daily basis and also meant Dad would see a familiar face he trusted every day.

I worked tirelessly to better the communication and trust between staff and family members at the facility. I learned to never take any caregiving issue for granted. If I didn't get the answers I needed, I went straight to the top of the management chain. Realizing I was my father's voice empowered me to do anything on his behalf.

Being involved in a caregivers group helped me know I wasn't alone and that others had issues similar to the ones I was having with my father. They were also able to offer helpful suggestions.

As an adopted child, it was good to be able to help, and care for, my father. It was a great way to pay him back for the great life he gave me.

♡

CONNIE'S JOURNEY: Terrified the Money was Going To Run Out

My mother was convinced for years that she had Alzheimer's. I didn't see any evidence of it but she was so scared that, when she was 80 years old, she went through a battery of tests. The tests confirmed she didn't have Alzheimer's but, since Mom was in Connecticut and I was in New York, I arranged for someone to come in anyway.

At first, Mom fought the idea but I told her it was just a companion for her and, before long, she fell in love with her "companion," Michele. They cooked together and Michele even took Mom line dancing. Michele had such a wonderful way with my mother and she became a very dear friend to my mother.

Mom always liked to cook but, since Michele wasn't coming every day, Mom was still cooking on her own. One day, Mom put a small pot of soup on the stove and forgot about it. Since she didn't have a sense of smell, she couldn't smell it smoldering and, before long, it caught fire. Gratefully, Mom was able to put out the fire but I got her a fire extinguisher and stopped her from unsupervised cooking. After that, I also had Michele come in every day.

Mom had an electric coffee percolator and a microwave so she could still cook small things but what really helped was that, when Michele was there, the two of them cooked up a storm. They cooked so much that, after Michele left, there was nothing else Mom needed (or wanted) to cook.

A few years later, Mom began to wane and started seeing her

therapist and doctor more often. Together, the therapist and doctor changed Mom's diagnosis to Alzheimer's.

Years before her diagnosis, Mom had looked at life-care centers and nursing homes. But she looked at them like you look at peas on a plate: you see them but you're not really interested; it's not something you really want. That's how it was for my mother — she looked at them but was completely adamant she didn't want to go into a nursing home.

My stepfather had died and left my mother with a reasonable trust but I was terrified the money was going to run out. Financial concerns and decisions are very different if you know you need money for two weeks, two months, two years or ten years. If you have this finite pot of money and the doctor says your parent won't live out the year, you don't worry about things. But there was no way to know how long we needed the money to last so I started thinking about things like reverse mortgages. I also got a geriatric care manager in Connecticut who was able to bring expenses into check.

Up to this point, Mom still lit up when I came to the door. She'd go in and out of recognition and ask me, "Where's Connie?" but if I kept telling her, "Mom, it's me" she'd eventually get it. But now, she didn't recognize me. Not at all. There wasn't even a glimmer of recognition. I could say she was completely "out of it" mentally but I don't know if that's true. Mom may have been mentally "out of it" from my perspective but she may have still been in there having thoughts.

Then Michele left to go to nursing school and we had a number of different caregivers. Eventually, we got a wonderful woman from Ghana who took exquisite care of my mother but, unfortunately, she hurt her back and her doctor said she couldn't continue caring for my mother.

After that, we went through a bunch of different geriatric care managers and caregivers. I didn't know what to do. It was like a revolving door of caregivers. We got blessed by some; others were nightmares. The other thing I didn't know was if it was going to be Mom's final month.

When Mom's physician noticed a bedsore, hospice was called in to examine Mom and, after that, hospice nurses came in every day. They became concerned over the revolving door of caregivers so, even though they were only supposed to come in to visit, treat Mom and leave, they spent hours with her until a nurse showed up.

One day I got a call from the hospice nurse saying they had noticed a bruise on my mother's upper thigh and were calling my mother's physician. The doctor told them to call an ambulance and have her taken to the hospital. Mom had a broken femur.

Connecticut Elder Services conducted an investigation but we still don't know exactly what happened. The best case scenario is that Mom was so fragile the bone broke when her caregiver was moving her and it wasn't intentional. The worse case is they were rough with Mom. I like to believe the best case scenario because anything else is unbearable.

I learned hospice was considering filing an abuse report with Elder Care — not against me, but against the agency that sent the caregiver. I'm a grown woman and an attorney yet, in that moment, I reverted back to being a child. It was like I was five years old. All I could think was that I was responsible for my mother's care and somehow the police were going to come and I was going to get arrested for being a bad daughter. I know that's completely irrational but at the time it was my initial response.

In the meantime, they were getting ready to discharge Mom from the hospital. Hospice suggested I consider having her discharged directly to a nursing home. I wanted to vomit. But then, after my initial reaction, it became clear to me that Mom would get stable care in a nursing home. And that's what she deserved: stable care. Not a revolving door. Her getting stable care was more important than what I wanted.

Miraculously, the Lutheran Home in Southbury, Connecticut had a bed available and Mom moved in.

You will not get better care anywhere. I was bowled over by these people. It's like they are caring for their own parents. They support both the patient and the family. If I stepped out into the hall looking like I was going to cry, a nurse would swoop me up and hug me. They would give me tea and cookies in the middle of the night when I was sitting up with Mom.

I still didn't know what we were looking at time-wise. I knew it wasn't good — and that Mom wasn't good — but I was trying to figure out if we were looking at a couple of months, or years. I was trying to figure out if I had to sell her house. Hospice told me they didn't think it was going to be that long. I think, on some level, I expected it but hearing it was a very different thing.

Mom went into the nursing home on July 30th. I got a call on August 4th saying I should get there sooner rather than later. Mom stopped eating on August 8th and died nine days later.

I had spent all that time worrying whether I'd have enough money to care for her. The money started to run out just before she passed away. But thank God it was there because that's what it was there for: to take care of my mother.

DAVID'S JOURNEY: The Wake-Up Call

My father was diagnosed with Alzheimer's in 2005. At the time, he was 77 years old, widowed, and living alone in Florida. I have two sisters: one in Houston and the other in Las Vegas. I had been living in Los Angeles but had recently moved to Kansas. My mom died ten years earlier but Dad didn't want to move closer to any of us. He wanted to stay in Florida.

This wasn't my first experience with Alzheimer's. Approximately 20 years earlier, my uncle had it and was living in a facility. There was a Hispanic gentleman named Reuben who worked at the facility and, when my cousin and I visited my uncle, I watched how Reuben was with the people in the facility. He remained positive and treated them with grace and humor. He humanized them and never got strung out by their condition or circumstances. Reuben was my first positive role model in how to deal with dementia and it helped me with my dad.

When I look back at how my father was diagnosed, it was a textbook case. I got a call from the police telling me my father was wandering around and didn't know where he was. Gratefully, there was an incident before that which had given me a head start.

In 2004, Florida was hit by four hurricanes. The area where Dad lived got direct hits from three of the hurricanes. After each one, I'd call and ask Dad how he was and he always assured me he was fine. After the third hurricane, I got a call from one of Dad's neighbors telling me I had to get down there because Dad's house was leaking, the rain was coming inside the house and that Dad was "living in a swamp."

I arrived the next day and found a severely damaged house. There were leaks everywhere, holes in the ceiling, the insulation was down, and the carpet was soaked. There was mold on the walls and the house smelled. Dad and his 10-year-old-dog, Mickey, were essentially sequestered to the one bedroom that didn't have any leaks.

I also found a father who was extremely confused and foggy. Dad hadn't bathed, was sleeping on dirty sheets, and was walking around in soiled, unwashed clothes. He seemed shell-shocked, disoriented and unable to process what had happened.

Since alcohol had always been a part of his (and our) life, I attributed his state of mind to advanced alcoholism. In hindsight, I believe it was a combination of alcohol, Alzheimer's, and the shock of the hurricanes and his subsequent living conditions.

On prior visits, I had taught Dad how to balance his checkbook and put various systems in place for him to pay bills. He'd always been able to shop for himself and enjoyed cooking so I was confident his bills were being paid and he was eating really well. There'd never been any signs otherwise. But this time I saw major slippage. I saw Dad was able to fake his way through phone conversations and convince people he was fine. When I looked over his paperwork and bills, I saw problems. He was eating very little and what he was eating was crap. This was my wake-up call.

I put a tarp on his roof in anticipation of the next hurricane which was projected to hit in a week. I cleaned up the soggy carpet and insulation, treated the mold on the wall, filed a FEMA claim, and left Dad in a more livable situation.

When I arrived back home, I immediately began researching Alzheimer's. I queried the Alzheimer's Association, searched for everything and anything relating to Alzheimer's and looked into Visiting Nurse and Meals on Wheels programs. In the midst of all of this, "the call" came.

Just before New Year's Eve, the phone rang and a police officer told me they'd found my father wandering in the next county.

The officer said my father apparently had been driving, got lost, never checked the fluids in his car and had essentially melted the engine. The officer also told me my father had been taken to the Winter Haven Hospital.

I called the hospital and every doctor and nurse I talked to told me they thought Dad either had dementia or Alzheimer's. They also said that legally they could only hold Dad for 72 hours and that I needed to contact Adult Protective Services. The possibility that our family could be accused of neglect added yet another dimension to the situation. I told them I'd be there the next day.

As soon as I arrived, I met with Adult Protective Services and learned that filing a claim was normal procedure but, nonetheless, I was happy to clear up any claim or assertion of neglect.

Gratefully, during my prior visit, I had met with Dad's attorney so all of his legal documents were in order to allow me to handle things.

I contacted the Alzheimer's Association and got leads on care facilities. I visited as many as possible and started getting Dad pre-approved for admission through his long-term critical care policy.

By this time, Dad had been in the hospital for five days and was detoxed from alcohol (a requirement for him to be admitted to any of the assisted living facilities).The doctor had also done an evaluation and declared Dad incompetent.

The best information I got the entire time was from a good friend who had gone through this with her father. She helped me sort things out — both in my mind and on paper. It was difficult finding a paper trail since much of Dad's paperwork had been drenched, trashed or rendered useless from the water damage in his house. However, I was able to piece together that Dad's homeowner's insurance had expired so he no longer had coverage for the damage to his home. I also discovered his property taxes were delinquent.

While Dad had medical insurance and a long-term critical care policy, I was still concerned whether there would be enough money to pay for his care so I filed a claim with the Veterans Administration.

I re-roofed and sold his house. Then I cleaned and emptied it, keeping whatever mementos I thought my sisters or I might want and giving some to neighbors who had done so much for Dad. I had a garage sale and whatever was left went to Goodwill.

The hardest thing I had to do was find a home for his dog, Mickey. Mickey had been Dad's companion since Mom died and I was worried not having her around would affect his mental state. I was able to find a wonderful home for Mickey. As it turned out, Dad never remembered her and never asked about her again. That was mind-boggling to me.

Dad was released from the hospital directly into Savannah Cottage, an amazing facility where the people really went out of their way to ensure Dad's care and comfort.

I don't think caring for a parent with Alzheimer's is beyond the capability of most people if you are willing to ask for support, get referrals and move step by logical step. One thing I would recommend is that people put on a thicker skin in order to motor through the logistics of caregiving. I have a great deal of heart and compassion but when it came to doing the things that needed to be done, I allowed my drill instructor side to come out. I'm proud of what I accomplished and the care my dad received.

♡

LESLIE'S JOURNEY: You Name It, Alzheimer's Took It

I'm 31 years old and single mother to a precious girl named Kierra. My older brother and I were raised by our mother after our father passed away. My mother was in her late 60s when she was diagnosed with Alzheimer's although there were signs before that.

Mom was always a hard worker, very fun-loving and extremely intelligent. Since she was always a wee bit "spacey" it was easy to ignore the first signs of Alzheimer's — things like misplacing her keys, losing her purse, or errors in the checkbook. Since the incidents were few and far between they were easy to ignore and, had it not been for our family history with Alzheimer's, I think I would have ignored the signs even longer.

Mom and I were best friends and very close. In 2001, when

Mom moved in with me to help me care for my newborn daughter, I began to notice changes in her personality. We began to argue about weird things. We'd argued before, but it was different now. She was angrier. She was also forgetting to eat, how to cook and had started losing a lot of weight. She was a small woman to begin with so losing any weight wasn't a good thing for her.

Mom had always been very friendly and patient but now she started getting snippy with people. She would get annoyed at store clerks, friends, and things my daughter did. She kept misplacing things and arguing with me. As her personality continued to change, I became more concerned.

But then Mom would do really well for several months and I would tell myself she was fine. Deep down, Mom knew what was happening but, like me, she didn't want to know and didn't want others to know either. She became a master at hiding what was going on.

I began researching Alzheimer's but kept the information to myself. However, on a trip to visit family in Canada, my aunt (who was caring for another aunt with Alzheimer's), noticed the signs and suggested we see a neurosurgeon.

Mom did a good job of covering up any problems she was having with the doctor but the MRI showed debris in her brain. She began getting monthly shots of Vitamin B12 and began taking Namenda. For a while, she did much better. Occasionally, she would have a bad day but the bad days came and went.

Then, one day, Mom got lost while taking my daughter for a walk. When the police found them, both my mom and daughter were covered in sweat and dehydrated. Mom blamed it on the heat and, since I was still trying to convince myself that Mom was fine, I agreed it probably was just the heat. It sounds crazy now but I loved her and, even though I knew what was happening, it was killing me to admit it. Even though I knew people would understand, I didn't want anyone to think less of her. My mother was my best friend and I just wasn't ready to admit it to myself.

By the end of 2004, I left my full-time job and, instead, took on two part-time jobs. One of my part-time jobs was at a local retirement home which was, in part, a blessing because I was learning a lot about Alzheimer's and the healthcare system. However, the downside was that I was dealing with Alzheimer's all day and then going home to it at night.

Since my hours at both jobs were inconsistent, Mom was being left alone more and more. I knew it was wrong but I was doing the best I could. I was also handling all of Mom's banking and other personal business by this time.

A few months later, things went from bad to worse — fast. Mom started hallucinating and became very paranoid and somewhat aggressive. To this day, I fear it was my work schedule that pushed her over the edge.

I was an emotional basket case. My brother lived across the country and when Mom got on the phone with him she was able to cover up her illness and act like everything was fine. I was having a difficult time convincing him there was something wrong so I started documenting everything and letting him listen to voicemails Mom left me. And then the breaking point came.

I arrived at work one morning and got a call from Mom. She was hysterical and angry, telling me she wanted to go home and didn't appreciate being left with a child she didn't even know.

I left work immediately and got my daughter into full-time daycare. We started Mom on medication for anxiety and hallucinations and got the Agency on Aging, as well as Health & Human Services, involved.

Mom was sundowning and would get very agitated at night and start pacing. I would fall asleep and Mom would wake me up wanting to know what she should be doing. One night she woke me up, irate, telling me it was inappropriate for me to be sleeping in her home. She threatened to call the police if I didn't leave. I started yelling at her hysterically and gave her the phone but, thankfully, she didn't call.

As Mom got worse, I got more and more stressed. I wanted the best for Mom. I wanted her to be somewhere where she wouldn't be alone and would have activities. I wanted to be able to visit her and be patient with her. I also knew I couldn't handle her any longer so Mom moved into a memory supported assisted living facility. The staff was amazing, her weight increased, and she improved a great deal.

The hardest part was when Mom cried and asked me why I was leaving her there. She wanted to go home and wanted to know what she had done to upset me and why I didn't want to live with her anymore.

Eventually, she settled in and the next few years were pretty good. Mom seemed happy and she wasn't alone.

The staff was great and did their best to respect the residents and treat them with dignity but it would have killed my mother — a once proud and beautiful woman — to know she needed help with every aspect of her life.

Alzheimer's stole my mother's life. It took everything from her — her pride, her health, her ability to care for herself, her memories, everything. It stole my mom, a Nana, a friend, happiness. You name it; Alzheimer's took it.

PAM'S JOURNEY: No Doubt The Alcohol Greatly Worsened the Disease

My mother and I first noticed changes in my father in 1997 after he retired. Retirement was a lifestyle upgrade for my parents. They moved to a nicer town and bigger house but, virtually overnight, Dad became anxious and unproductive. He followed Mom from room to room, fussing and worrying as they set up their new house. It took him months and months to settle down.

Three years before Dad retired — and after a lifetime of total sobriety — my parents had suddenly started drinking. So I was worried about my dad's memory loss but also about my parents' drinking.

My husband is a physician and he agreed there was cause for concern. I spoke with my brothers but they both dismissed my concerns. The only other family I could talk to were aunts and cousins but, again, no one wanted to talk to my parents and, since I didn't dare confront them alone, nothing was ever said.

I was living in Delaware and, since my parents were living in Canada, it was difficult to do anything. I saw them every few months but spoke with them almost every day. I noticed Dad, who had always been an articulate speaker, had begun to paraphrase more and was struggling to find the right words. He also seemed apathetic and unmotivated.

In the summer of 2003, my husband and I had to return to his native country to resolve a visa problem, which required us to live abroad for two years. So, just as my concerns about my parents were increasing, even more distance was put between us.

I had convinced myself that Dad had alcohol-related dementia and, if he stopped drinking, he would regain some of his memory. When my parents visited us overseas, I decided to express my concerns about their drinking and Dad's memory loss. My father refused to acknowledge a drinking problem and was shocked over my concerns about his memory.

My mother, on the other hand, apologized profusely and seemed genuinely grateful I had been willing to broach these difficult subjects. However, even though she handled it well that day, she became angry afterwards and treated me with hostility for almost a year. I was afraid she'd never forgive me.

Since I was still living outside the country, I don't know the exact chronology of the events that followed. I know at some point after our conversation, Dad went to see a neurologist who tested him for dementia and, while he didn't give him a diagnosis, he did start him on medication (presumably the Aricept and Namenda that he takes to this day).

From far away in Europe, I tried to get my dad to exercise, stop eating like a bird, stop drinking like a fish, get involved in their new community, and (most of all) to fight against his slide into oblivion. I was mad at him for a long time because he didn't do anything to fight it but I now understand that Alzheimer's stole my dad's initiative long before it stole his vocabulary.

We are currently using a social service agency. We were floored by the cost but they have been helpful in finding a better doctor, safety-proofing their home, and chipping away at my mother's denial.

I have a lot of regrets about not getting my family to address the drinking problem when it first emerged. While I know my dad doesn't have alcohol-related dementia there is no doubt in my mind that the alcohol greatly worsened his illness.

It has taken Dad ten years to get to early stage four but I can't help thinking he wouldn't be like this if he hadn't been drinking. He wouldn't call my daughter "little girl" because he would know her name is Sarah; he wouldn't scare my son with his obsessions; and he wouldn't put my children's lives in danger by trying to put them in the car and take them for a ride.

I tried to intervene in my parents' alcohol consumption but it had little to no effect. The same thing is happening now with my father and driving. Despite my repeated attempts, no one in the family is willing to take an active role with this problem. Once again, I'm alone in the battle. No one will help me. I don't know what to do. My parents act like I'm the enemy but I live in eternal fear that he'll kill or maim someone's child.

♡

RHONDA'S JOURNEY: "Maybe...maybe...maybe..."

My mother was born in Belgium, as was my biological father, although I haven't seen him since I was 21. My parents separated when I was ten and my sister was eight. Up until then, our lives had seemed pretty Ozzie and Harriet.

At the time my parents separated, my mom was fairly crippled with arthritis but she still went to work by opening a second-hand shop in Santa Cruz with her best friend, April. An artist and antiques dealer named Bob had a booth nearby. Eventually, Bob and my mom fell in love and got married on Valentine's Day. Of all the people I know, they are the only two I can honestly call soulmates. When they are together, it's like the rest of the world doesn't exist.

Not long after they were married, Bob adopted my sister and me and we all moved to California. However, we were struggling financially so we decided to move once again. This time we moved, not just out of the state, but out of the country to what was, at the time, the cheapest country to live in: Spain.

We sold everything — including some masterpieces Bob had

painted — and our family spent the next five years in Spain. Through it all, Bob and I became very close and I began to call him Dad.

Mom's arthritis had gotten much worse. She'd been told she would be in a wheelchair within a few years but Dad nurtured my mother back to health with love. After a few years, they were walking on the beaches of Spain holding hands, my mother showing no trace of the disease.

Dad's paintings were selling faster than he could paint them. He also entered, and won, a worldwide art competition. He was the first American to ever win the competition and was invited to Brussels for a black tie dinner with the King and Queen of Belgium, where Dad was given a title and medal.

My brother was born while we were in Spain and he became the new joy in our lives. Those were good years. When rumors began circulating that civil war might erupt in Spain, we decided it was time to go. We moved back to the States, to North Carolina, where my parents opened a small antiques shop.

High school graduation, college, marriages, babies and divorces followed. Then, ten years ago, Dad, who was always brilliant, began forgetting things. Our initial thought was maybe it was a mini-stroke, or maybe clogged arteries, or maybe he was tired. Maybe...maybe...maybe...until, at last, we received a diagnosis: dementia. Five years later, the diagnosis was changed to Alzheimer's.

When I shared Dad's diagnosis with a close friend he said, "You have no idea what you're in for. There's no way to describe it. You'll experience a pain no one can prepare you for and you'll experience a hell unlike anything you've ever read or heard about. And I'll be here for you through it all."

I thought my friend was simply being dramatic.

Even though the changes came on ever-so-subtly, it was obvious the disease was progressing and that my dad was beginning the journey away from us. He knew it and so did we. He would say, "Nothing's wrong. I'm fine. I didn't forget anything" but there it was taking him, little by little, every day. And there was nothing any of us could do to stop it.

Since Dad was an artist, we measured the disease's progress

through his work. Every time he came down from his studio with a painting, we let out a collective sigh. But then he started going upstairs to his studio to work and, over and over, would come back down empty-handed. He would say he wasn't motivated or the light wasn't right or the room was too hot. He was trying to spare us from the truth and we all tried living in denial until we simply couldn't deny it any longer.

One day my mother called me. She was crying so hard she couldn't speak so I got in my car and drove over to their house. When I arrived, Mom was still in tears. "He came downstairs and told me he was finished with this," she said, holding up a painting. My dad had been a master of trompe l'oeil. He had the ability to make things look so real you thought you were looking at a photograph. In the painting my mother was holding, Dad hadn't finished the background and the pot of tulips was completely out of perspective — yet he had signed it just as he'd done with every other one of his creations. Before I could say anything, my dad came around the corner, "Do you like it?" he asked.

"Yeah Dad, I love it."

I stayed and had a cup of coffee with him, then I got in my car and drove home, sobbing.

There were two years when Daddy was keenly aware of what was happening and I think those were the hardest years for him. He had always known the words to all of the operas (in both Italian and French) and knew about antiques, paintings, prints and lithographs. He restored artwork and was a brilliant painter. But the brilliance was escaping. We tried pills. We tried mind games and board games and computer games to challenge him mentally. We talked to him for hours and asked him questions to keep his mind working but Dad continued to slip away. Alzheimer's was an impossible enemy to combat.

Since Dad no longer spoke our language, I tried some of the techniques I use to teach children who speak other languages to reach him. By simplifying language, it helped communication between us and Mom said, at the time, I was able to reach him at a level no one else could.

Then the disease stole his memories of my children and the following year, his memories of me vanished.

After my brother's wife died, he moved in with my parents. My dad hasn't known my brother for several years and every day the situation grows worse. My dad believes my brother is a stranger who has come into his house to steal from him.

Recently, Dad's body has begun to give out. He has long since forgotten how to wash the dishes, open a can or find things in the kitchen. He no longer knows how to lift the toilet seat, dress himself in proper clothes, or wash himself.

Mom no longer sleeps through the night because Dad wanders. They have alarms on the door that stop him from going out (assuming he would even know how to turn the key to get out). On the rare occasion he does sleep, he wets the bed.

My sister found a day program through the Veterans Administration so now, when Dad's at the program, Mom sleeps if she can — only to start all over again when he comes home.

Mom had a part-time job to bring in extra income, keep her sanity and find a reason to pull herself together in the morning but now she's had to stop working. I've watched my mother age in these last few months and now I'm afraid my mother is the one who's dying.

I tell Mom it's time to find a place for Daddy but she says he took care of her when she couldn't walk and now it's her turn to care for him.

♡

SHIRLEY'S JOURNEY: That One Day Changed Everything

My father, Robert, was diagnosed with Alzheimer's when he was 75 years old — although the symptoms started before that. The initial diagnosis was made based on his shuffling gait, loss of memory, paranoia, and accusations of theft.

I was 43, widowed, a mother and working full-time when my father was diagnosed. I'm the oldest of three children and my parents were living on the family farm about two and a half hours from my home.

My younger brother, Donald, lived with my parents in the big farmhouse. When he got married, he and his wife stayed in the farmhouse and my parents moved next door into a cottage. In those days, Dad was still able to go to the barn and feed the calves and unload wagons. Most days, you could never tell there was a problem.

Unlike some families who keep an Alzheimer's diagnosis from their loved one, my father knew. My mother felt keeping it from him would rob them of their marriage vows to love one another "for better or worse, for richer or poorer, in sickness and in health." Plus, my parents had always trusted and been completely honest with each other.

Early on, my father didn't deny his fears or insecurities about the future but, when the disease progressed, he began to vehemently deny the diagnosis. He went through a long period of struggle, alternately accepting and denying his diagnosis.

I think part of it was that my father understood what the diagnosis meant for him in the long run because his younger brother, Clair, had been diagnosed with early-onset Alzheimer's. My aunt had taken care of my uncle at home until he became physically violent towards her. After that, my uncle was transferred to an Alzheimer's unit at a veterans hospital. It nearly broke my aunt's heart. She loved my uncle and visited him every day.

As we continued getting updates about my uncle, my father wrestled with whether or not he wanted to visit his brother. Part of his concern was not knowing what to say or do during the visit; the other, I believe, was because facing his brother was, in a sense, looking at his own future. My father, once so self-assured and certain, was in such personal conflict. It was painful to watch and was one of the most difficult things I ever witnessed my father go through.

A couple of years went by and, finally, my father and mother decided to visit my uncle. Even though they knew it was going to be difficult, I think my father needed to say goodbye to his younger brother. I held out hope my uncle would recognize my dad or, at the very least, they'd be able to talk about something from their childhood.

When my parents arrived, they found my uncle in a wheelchair, looking the picture of health. However, he was talking nonsense and didn't recognize my father or mother. My parents didn't stay very long and while I believe the visit gave my father some closure, it also left him with a very vivid image of what he would become. My father kept saying, "He looked perfectly healthy. If you met him on the street you would never know anything was wrong." My father never spoke about the visit, or his brother, after that and, six months later, my uncle died.

My mother took care of my father but, as time passed, my mother's health began to deteriorate. She underwent numerous surgeries, including heart bypass surgery. My brother and sister-in-law, along with my son and me, all helped out and even though Dad's illness was progressing, it was all still manageable until the accident.

In March 2002, my parents were involved in a horrific single car accident and they were both airlifted to a hospital. My mother was seriously injured and was placed in an induced coma in intensive care for almost one month. My father suffered a fractured rib and broken neck vertebrae but, miraculously, hadn't severed his spinal cord. He, too, was placed in intensive care but in a separate part of the hospital from Mom. He desperately wanted to be with her but that was impossible.

After two weeks in the hospital, Dad's insurance company demanded he be sent for rehabilitation. My brothers and I didn't want to put Dad in a rehab facility but we didn't have any other viable options at the time. None of us were prepared to care for Dad at home and, even though he had long-term care insurance, the waiting period hadn't passed. We had two days' notice to put a plan into place. The hospital's social services were terrific but we had to battle with Dad's insurance company to place him in a facility near his home.

My brothers and I had concerns over the care Dad was receiving in the rehab facility but we felt powerless to do much about it. We were at a total loss as to how to navigate the system and to reliably review our options. There was also a great deal of confusion because none of us knew our parents' financial situation.

As soon as Dad was moved, he began to rapidly deteriorate—mentally and physically — and, eventually, he had to be moved into a separate Alzheimer's unit at the facility.

My mother fought her way back but, to a large degree, was

permanently wounded by the accident. It destroyed her sense of security and she became obsessed with finances. Even though my parents had medical insurance, the bills we received on their behalf were staggering and my mother started making decisions based solely on what things cost rather than on quality-of-life.

It was the second worst episode in my life. The first was my husband and son's accident but that, I firmly believe, helped prepare me for this part of my life. But still everyone was numb — my brothers, myself, my parents' siblings, the community in which they lived — everyone. That one day changed everything.

SYLVIA'S JOURNEY: I Want To Love and Care for Him the Best I Can

My father has Alzheimer's. Even though he hasn't had an official diagnosis, our family knows it's Alzheimer's. We don't need a doctor to tell us.

My sister and sister-in-law are both registered nurses and they handle the medical-related issues. My brother and other sister handle the finances. My youngest brother does what he can. And I'm now the live-in caregiver for both of my parents.

I had been living in Kansas and my siblings had been taking care of both of my parents for quite a while. Three of my four siblings have families and they had a lot on their plates. We all knew it was best if someone lived with my parents since there were a lot of things that weren't being tended to but none of them wanted to ask me to come back. I always knew I would come back one day to help and they were happy when I did.

It took me a good four months to adjust to being back. I didn't want to be there. I felt confined. I lost all my freedom. I had no privacy. And I felt guilty for feeling like that. I met other people who were caregivers and they handled it with such apparent ease and grace and I felt I should be able to do it, too.

It was very difficult being back in my parents' house as an adult. Our lifestyles and ideologies are different and we are at opposite ends of the spectrum when it comes to religion and politics. I've also never had a regular 40-hour-a-week job. I've either been self-employed or worked part-time. I'm creative and have an artistic temperament, so I need alone time. I'm struggling to find the time and space to muse, dream, create, socialize, or just be outside in Nature.

Initially, I felt like I was on call all the time because I live with my parents. Over time, I came to realize I needed to get out of the house on a regular basis. Since my parents need the most help in the morning and evening, I take time in the afternoon for myself. I have to leave the house though because, if I'm around, they want me with them so I go to a coffee shop and write, I meet a friend for lunch or I just take a walk or sit in the park. I don't feel quite so overwhelmed now.

When I first moved home, Dad was in the early stages of Alzheimer's. Back then, Mom's health was worse than Dad's so my main focus was on helping Mom as well as cooking meals, cleaning and doing all the things they couldn't do. But then we began to notice Dad was having trouble and now, one year later, I see him declining noticeably from one month to the next. I watch Dad losing his abilities, cognition and independence. He asks a question or tells us something and then repeats himself two minutes later. It used to be maybe a couple hours, or days, but now he literally doesn't remember from one minute to the next. The decline is escalating — and I feel so helpless to stop it.

My dad is an outgoing, gregarious, cheerful, fun-loving man. He was always the life of the party and very social but now I see he is losing his friends. His social circle is getting smaller and smaller. People who used to go out of their way to visit him are staying away. I think they're embarrassed for him, they don't know how to react, or they don't like hearing the same story, or being asked the same question, over and over.

Well-meaning people have suggested we give Dad little jobs around the house, but he's unable to do even the simplest task. He can't load the dishwasher or take out the trash out anymore. Sometimes if I ask him to do something, he'll wander around the room with a blank look on his face like he doesn't know what I mean or where to begin. He's constantly misplacing things and if I tell him where they are, he'll walk around looking but he seems to have lost the ability to follow or understand directions.

Going forward, I have some very real concerns. The first would be if Mom died first (which is a possibility considering her health). If that happened, I believe Dad would decline very rapidly. After 52 years together, they've become very dependent on one another. Also, Dad would no longer be able to live alone. I believe he would do very well in an assisted living situation because he's so active and social and there would be people around. I yearn for him to be somewhere where he can walk down the hall and visit with friends but he thinks those places are for "old people" — not for him. He wants to stay in the house he built.

I'm also concerned that Dad is still driving. Mom isn't physically able to drive so she goes along in the car and directs him. They do okay but he's very slow on his left-hand turns. We haven't wanted to take driving away from him too, because we live in an area where there is no public transportation. It would drive Dad crazy to be in the house all day.

I don't ever remember my father getting angry when I was growing up. Since Alzheimer's, I see him getting angry more often. It may have to do with frustration or a loss of control because he was always the one in charge. Now he doesn't always make appropriate decisions and, if we question or correct him, he gets angry. Dad is a big man and extremely strong. I've heard that sometimes people with this disease can get violent and I worry what we would do if that ever happened.

My other concern is that, because he's so physically robust, his mind will continue to deteriorate but he'll live a long, long, long time. That would be sad.

But mostly my concerns are about loving and caring for my father to the best of my ability. He's so sweet and really is a good man. I was thinking recently that I wasn't focusing as much attention on him as I should so when he was outside I went out by him and said, "I just want to hug you and tell you I love you." I need to do more of that.

The First Steps on Your Journey

Whether your parent was recently diagnosed — or you've been caring for your parent for years — the unpredictable nature of Alzheimer's can cause uncertainty and a lack of confidence in any caregiver. You may be unsure where to begin, what to do first (or next) and where to turn for help.

I asked caregivers, based on their personal experience, the following question:

"If a good friend told you their parent had just been diagnosed with Alzheimer's, what would you tell them are the first steps they should take?"

Here is what they said:

YOUR FIRST STEPS
1. Get a Diagnosis — and the Right Doctor
2. Get Your Family Together
3. Get Support
4. Get Your Legal and Financial Affairs in Order

In the following pages, you will meet additional caregivers and hear, in greater detail, why they recommend the above steps.

You will also learn that you *can* do this. As exhausted, overwhelmed or unsure as you may be right now, you'll begin to see that — while it won't always be easy and you can't do it alone — you *can* do this by taking it one day, and one step, at a time.

Before we begin, I'd like to share one very special reply I received to the above question since it provides a unique, and sometimes unspoken, perspective.

> *I would tell my friend the first thing they need to do is to still be there for their parent and support them because your parent needs you now more than ever. Second, I would tell them to contact their local Alzheimer's chapter for support and advice. And, the last thing I would tell them is that there is life **after** an Alzheimer's diagnosis. I would tell them to encourage their parent to continue to be as active as possible to keep their brain stimulated. The old saying is true: "Use it or lose it."*
>
> *I hope it's okay that I answered this question. I'm not a caregiver but the person with dementia. — Tracy*

STEP #1: Get a Diagnosis and the Right Doctor

We'll begin by asking an obvious question: "Has your mother (or father) been diagnosed with Alzheimer's?" If not, caregivers say that is your first — and most important — step.

Get A Diagnosis

Even though your parent may be growing more forgetful and, while you believe you *know* it's Alzheimer's, until you hear the words come out of a trusted doctor's mouth, you really *don't* know. There are other illnesses and diseases whose symptoms mimic Alzheimer's. Schedule a complete and thorough exam for your parent and make sure you know exactly what you're dealing with.

At the initial exam, be prepared to provide the doctor with the following:

- ❑ Your parent's medical history (if the doctor doesn't already have that information).
- ❑ Symptoms you, your parent or your family have noticed, when they began, their frequency and if they are getting worse.
- ❑ Family medical history and, in particular, if any other family members had (or has) Alzheimer's or other form of dementia.
- ❑ Medication your parent is currently taking (including dosage and frequency).

Since there currently isn't a single test that can conclusively diagnose Alzheimer's, the doctor may run a series of tests and also refer your parent to a neurologist or other specialist for further testing and evaluation.

Many caregivers say getting a diagnosis was difficult since their parent was unwilling to accept there was anything wrong and felt a diagnosis was completely unnecessary. Due to doctor/patient confidentiality and restrictions under the HIPAA laws, it may be difficult (and, in some instances, unlawful) for you to discuss your parent's condition with their doctor unless your parent has given their doctor permission to do so.

One of our caregivers, Jaye, explained how she was able to get a diagnosis for her mother while still respecting the limits of the law.

> I suspected Mom was having problems for years. It wasn't just her forgetfulness but her personality and behavior were also changing. She worried about things — small things — to the point of obsession. She stopped driving. When I visited, I noticed she wasn't as social as she used to be and would stay close to my father, almost as if for security.
>
> I tried several times to talk with my father but, for his own reasons, he didn't (or couldn't) admit that anything

was wrong. I tried once to broach the subject with Mom but she said she had no idea what I was talking about so I just let it go.

Out of desperation, I decided to reach out to Mom's doctor. I liked and trusted him but I also knew, since Mom was otherwise healthy, she was only seeing him once (or maybe twice) a year. I also knew that during those visits, Mom was probably able to cover up any symptoms with a smile or a joke and that her doctor probably had no idea what was happening.

Since I don't live nearby, I sat down and wrote Mom's doctor a letter. I told him about the changes I'd seen in Mom's behavior and how long it had been happening. I knew, because of doctor /patient confidentiality laws, he couldn't discuss Mom's health with me, but I asked him to keep my comments in mind the next time he saw her.

A few weeks later, Dad said Mom's doctor called and asked her to come in for blood tests. The doctor had apparently taken my comments to heart since, while she was there, he did some cognition tests, too. The doctor told Mom she was probably in the early stages of Alzheimer's and recommended she begin taking Aricept. Dad said she was livid. I felt guilty because I felt I was the cause of her upset. But then I realized, now that we finally knew, it meant we could begin discussing how we were going to take care of Mom.

Jaye's mother's reaction to her diagnosis isn't that uncommon. Most caregivers say their parent was unable to accept the initial diagnosis. Some say the denial was only a temporary reaction; others say their parent initially accepted the diagnosis only to deny it later on. Still others say their parent never accepted the diagnosis.

How your parent processes the diagnosis may be determined by their belief system, their personality and how they handled crises in the past. Denial may have always been your parent's favorite coping strategy or they may believe (or want to believe) the doctor will somehow take care of the problem and everything will be fine.

Acceptance is a process. Give your parent the time, space and support they need to come to some level of acceptance of their diagnosis. If they don't, it's not up to you or anyone else to get your parent to accept the diagnosis. Your job is to love and support them on their journey with the disease.

———⟨◎⟩———

- We told Dad he was having "memory problems." We never used the Alzheimer's label with him. — *Allyson*

- My mother didn't accept the diagnosis and, honestly, it's not really something most people would want to accept. As much as possible, I just worked around her denial. — *Betsy*

- Even though I think he knew there was a problem, far be it for my father to admit it. He was always stubborn so refusing to accept the diagnosis was par for the course. — *Bill*

- We knew something was wrong with my mother-in-law but she refused to go to the doctor. It wasn't until she was violent and had to be taken to the hospital by the police that it was confirmed she did, indeed, have Alzheimer's. Those days before the diagnosis were difficult days. — *Chris*

- It may not be necessary (or sometimes even healthy) for the parent to accept a diagnosis of Alzheimer's. Some people give up and deteriorate rapidly when they are faced with a terminal diagnosis. In order to get them to take medication, if necessary, you (or their doctor) may wish to tell them it's something to "help their memory" or "keep them health." — *J. Lucy Boyd, RN, BSN*

- We never said the word "Alzheimer's" to Mom. We told her she had a mini-stroke which caused her dementia and, since she had been a nurse for over 30 years, she accepted her symptoms were side effects of the stroke. — *Judy*

- We never used the word "Alzheimer's" with my dad. He never wanted to know he had it and I was happy to indulge him that one small wish. — *Wanda*

———⟨◎⟩———

Get the Right Doctor

Having the right doctor on your journey is critical. The right doctor will become one of the most valuable members of your parent's caregiving team in the months and years to come. The right
doctor can alleviate (and possibly eliminate) problems and may
be able to help diffuse a future crisis for you or your parent.

The right doctor is one who is experienced with Alzheimer's,
knows how to deal with an Alzheimer's patient, and takes the
time to get to know your parent — as well as the rest of the family. The right doctor is one you, your parent, and your family,
respects and trusts.

If you don't currently have such a doctor (or team of doctors)
for your parent, take the time *now* to find one. Caregivers suggest:

- ❏ Asking friends, family, colleagues, support group members
  or organizations for referrals.
- ❏ Getting references.
- ❏ Checking the doctor's credentials.
- ❏ Meeting with the doctor — with, and if possible, without
  your parent.
- ❏ Trusting your instincts.

Frank, one of our caregivers, shared his experience of what
can happen if your parent doesn't have the right doctor.

*When my father was first diagnosed with Alzheimer's, we
had a family doctor we respected and trusted. He was
wonderful to Dad and understood Alzheimer's. He took
the time to talk with Dad, and the rest of the family, and
helped us put a plan together so Dad would always be
safe and well cared for.*

*Since the doctor understood Alzheimer's, he knew get-
ting Dad ready for appointments was difficult and that
time spent in the waiting room would only aggravate the
situation. Therefore, his staff brought Dad and my mom
(or sister) to an exam room as soon as they arrived. The
doctor was calm and respectful to Dad and, as a result,
appointments were without incident.*

Unfortunately, Dad's doctor had to retire due to his own health issues. We assumed his replacement would have the same level of integrity, compassion and understanding but we couldn't have been more wrong.

Before we met the new doctor for the first time, I faxed over a note briefly outlining Dad's history with Alzheimer's. On the day of the exam, I saw the fax sitting in Dad's file but it became obvious, within seconds, that the doctor had never taken the time to read it. He immediately began asking questions that upset Dad — and me.

Things didn't improve over time. The new doctor never got to know my father, the situation, or our family. He didn't care how long we waited for appointments. By the time we got into the examining room, Dad was often upset and agitated and the doctor couldn't get us out of there quick enough.

When Dad went through an angry phase and began to lash out verbally (especially at my mother), I took a leave of absence from my job to try and help my mother and sister. The first thing we did was call Dad's new doctor for advice. He never talked to us directly but, instead, had his nurse tell us the next time it happened to take Dad to the emergency room so they could adjust his medication.

A few days later, we followed the doctor's instructions. First, because Dad was already angry and agitated, it was an ordeal getting him into the car — but getting him out was even worse. It took five hospital employees and me over an hour to talk him out of the car; and he still went into the ER kicking and screaming. My mother, sister and I sat in the waiting area, filling out paperwork, and listening to Dad scream and curse. It was awful.

The ER doctor and Dad's new doctor told us they considered Dad to be a potential danger and, therefore, couldn't release him back to our care. They said Dad should be admitted to a psychiatric hospital so they could adjust his medications. None of us had any experience with this and, since we still trusted Dad's new doctor, we signed the papers and Dad was transferred. Honestly, we thought Dad would be there a few days, they'd get his medication adjusted, and we'd bring him back home. Again, we couldn't have been more wrong.

The first week, we weren't allowed to visit Dad in order to give him "time to adjust." The second week, we were allowed to visit but only twice a week and during very limited hours.

When we finally saw Dad, we were shocked. He was like a zombie. Strapped in a wheelchair, his head was slumped to one side and he was barely able to open his eyes. Dad had no idea my mother, my sister or I were there or who we were. We asked the nurses when he would be coming home and were told they had to stabilize Dad before he could be released.

Six weeks later, Dad was slightly more alert. He still didn't recognize my mother, my sister or me but the hospital said he was "stable." We were anxious to get Dad home but found out before they would release Dad back to our care, we had to appear before a State board to prove we were capable of caring for him.

I believe all of this could have been avoided if Dad's new doctor had simply taken the time to get to know Dad and our family and had become our partner in caring for Dad.

- Find a good doctor. Ask at local nursing homes or Alzheimer's facilities. — *Betsy*

- Get your parent to sign a HIPAA release form for every doctor so that you can stay informed of their progress and medication changes. — *Donna*

- Don't talk about the appointment too far in advance. Your parent might grow anxious or refuse to go. And when the day/time arrives for the appointment, stay calm, stay positive and talk about it matter-of-factly. Don't make a big deal about it. Also make sure the nurses and office staff know your parent has

Alzheimer's so they can assist in making sure visits go quickly and smoothly. — *Frank*

- Prepare a list of questions for the doctor and take notes so you can keep track of information or keep other family members updated. When the doctor asks a question, allow your parent to answer. This will help the doctor assess your parent. If possible, bring another person to assist you. This is particularly helpful at the end of the exam. One person can take your parent out to the waiting room or car while the other stays behind to talk with the doctor or pay the bill. — *Jaye*

- If you don't have complete faith in your doctor, keep looking. Get another opinion. Don't allow any doctor to write your parent off or over-medicate them. Find a geriatric physician or doctor you trust and have them review your parent's medications on a regular basis. — *Judy*

- Ask how they were diagnosed. General and family practitioners often diagnose Alzheimer's disease when there is a treatable condition with similar symptoms. Seek a second opinion by a neurologist. — *Kitty*

- Type up a list of any medications, vitamins and supplements your parent takes (including the name of the drug, dosage and frequency). Make copies for all family members. Keep it updated and with you at all times. It is helpful for doctor's appointments and extremely important if you ever have an emergency. — *Patti*

- Not all doctors or hospitals are created equal. Don't rely on your family physician or general practitioner for a diagnosis or continuing care for your parent. Seek out a specialist in Alzheimer's and ask for a geriatric assessment. Request family members attend. They will be provided with a lot of useful information and the professional may be able to mediate the family in meaningful dialogue (e.g. "Where do we go from here?"). — *Shirley*

- Get a thorough medical evaluation by a multi-specialty practice or neurologist who is familiar with Alzheimer's. Know what you're dealing with. — *Victoria*

STEP #2: Get Your Family Together

A diagnosis of Alzheimer's impacts every member of a family, and for that reason, your family may be your first — and most logical — line of defense and support.

Some caregivers say that talking with their family after the initial diagnosis was both helpful and healing. They say it helped establish open lines of communication and support and allowed them to discuss the diagnosis as well as their parent's present — and future — needs.

Other caregivers say it was extremely difficult for their family to discuss their parent's diagnosis, the future, or anything related to Alzheimer's.

Your family's ability to meet and talk will depend upon the personalities, relationships and dynamics that exist within your family. For some families, the idea of talking about your parent's diagnosis — and future — may be as natural as breathing; for others, it may be extraordinarily difficult, if not impossible. Your family may have never had a discussion — or any discussion — like this before. Family members may also be struggling with a variety of emotions — including grief.

People typically think of grief in the context of losing someone who has died but we all experience loss — and therefore grief — at various times throughout our lives. We may experience grief when we sell a much-loved car, or move from a comfortable place, house or job. People go through a grief process when they retire, or when their children start kindergarten, go off to college, or get married. We grieve what is left behind or what we knew — regardless of how excited we may be about the future.

Grief encompasses an entire experience — a cluster of feelings, thoughts, sensations and behaviors — that people go through when losing something or someone. In 1969, Dr. Elizabeth Kübler-Ross wrote a remarkable book titled *On Death and Dying* in which she defines the stages of grief: Denial, Anger, Guilt, Sadness, and Acceptance. This grief process, as described by Dr. Kübler-Ross, is what your parent, you and other family members may experience beginning with the initial diagnosis.

If diagnosed in the early stages, your parent may be aware enough to experience their own loss and grief. They may know what lies ahead and aware of what they will be losing. They may become depressed, despondent, withdrawn and fearful.

After a diagnosis, it is not uncommon for an entire family to be thrown into an ongoing cycle of loss and anxiety. As the disease progresses, it becomes an emotional roller coaster that takes us towards acceptance one minute then dashes us downward toward denial or depression the next. Feelings of loss are riddled with heightened fear of the unknown thereby making the grieving process an ongoing one.

Since every family member is unique, they will each face, and come to terms with, the reality of the disease in their own way. Everyone is hurting, everyone is suffering some kind of loss, yet everyone is experiencing the loss differently. This individual process of acceptance and grieving is usually the reason behind conflicts or misunderstandings between family members.

Patricia Fares–O'Malley, PhD. is a psychologist, educator and international speaker. She is also a Bereavement Coordinator for hospice and the author of "Healing The Love Wound."

If conflict or emotions are running high, you may be tempted to avoid, skip, or postpone getting your family together until things have calmed down or everyone is at the same level of acceptance. However, consider that:

- things may never calm down.
- there may never come a point where everyone is at the same level of acceptance.
- avoiding or delaying making decisions could drastically change your family's future — and the future care your parent receives.

The sooner your family comes together, the sooner you can begin developing a plan to love and care for your parent. Avoiding the discussion could mean going forward without a plan and spending the coming months — and years — reacting to crisis after crisis and hoping for a successful outcome. Not the best, or healthiest, solution for anyone — especially your parent.

Should I Include My Parent in the Discussion?

Whether you include your parent in the initial family discussion or meeting is a very personal decision. Because their parent was still in denial over their diagnosis, some caregivers say it wasn't possible to include them. Some were concerned the family would discuss things that might upset their parent so they chose not to include them. Some caregivers say, after hearing their family's plan for their future care, it enabled their parent to move to a new level of acceptance regarding their diagnosis.

Ultimately, your decision will be based on your best judgment as well as your understanding of your parent, your family and family dynamics.

If your family decides to include your parent in the family meeting, allow them to speak first. Listen to what your parent says — and what they don't — and watch their body language. Allowing your parent to talk first may enlighten everyone as to their wishes for their future — and future care. You may find your parent's wishes are quite different from what you thought they wanted. Hearing your parent's wishes first-hand also takes some of the guesswork out of what to do and allows your family to put a plan together based on your parent's needs and wishes.

It's important for all family members to understand that, unless it's a matter of safety or your parent has been declared incompetent, your parent has the right to make decisions regarding their life and care. Even if you don't agree with your parent's wishes, once you know them your family's job is to understand and do everything possible to support them. Remember, first and foremost, this disease is impacting your parent. Their life is slipping away. Allow your parent a voice, and the ability to maintain as much control as possible over their life, for as long as possible.

> As soon as Dad was diagnosed, our parents suggested we have a family meeting. Some of us were comfortable with the idea, others not so much, but because we were all committed to Dad's care, even those who were resistant jumped on board.
>
> At our initial meeting, we allowed Dad to talk first, then Mom. From that, we saw what his, her and their

concerns and needs were and allowed us to put a plan together to address them. I think both of our parents relaxed knowing their wishes were going to be respected and that their family was going to work together to care for and support them. — Frank

SUGGESTIONS FOR FAMILY MEETINGS

❏ Limit participants to close relatives (or immediate family). A maximum of seven or eight people will make the meeting more manageable.

❏ If possible, meet face-to-face in a comfortable, neutral location. If geographical location makes meeting in person impossible, schedule a conference call.

❏ Some family members, especially if they are resistant to the idea, may find every suggested day/time inconvenient. Set a time that is convenient for most and continue to invite and encourage any resistant family member(s) to participate.

❏ Any long-standing difficulties between family members need to be shelved. This meeting is about your parent. It is not a time to air, or rehash, old grievances and grudges as doing so will only further upset your parent.

❏ If your family is uncertain how to conduct the meeting (or if you're concerned that long-standing grudges might surface), consider using a mediator. A mediator should be a neutral party — perhaps a trusted friend, advisor or professional — rather than a family member. The mediator can moderate your discussion, keep an eye on the time, avoid interruptions, ensure that everyone stays on topic and keep the lines of communication open. If possible, all family members should agree on the choice of mediator and divide the cost of his/her fee in order for the mediator to be viewed as a neutral party and eliminate any concern they are affiliated or siding with a particular family member.

❏ Prepare and, if possible, agree on an agenda in advance.

❏ Establish basic rules of courtesy and respect — such as not interrupting when someone is speaking.

❏ Allow each family member adequate time to share their opinions and concerns without dominating the meeting. Consider using a timer and give each person an allotted time to speak.

❏ Ask everyone to come to the meeting with three or four specific concerns. Ask the mediator (or a family member) to write down the concerns and, when you have a complete list, decide on their order of urgency.

❑ Begin brainstorming ideas for your concerns, starting with the most urgent.

❑ If the list is too lengthy, or people's energy and focus are waning, end the meeting. Pick up where you left off at your next meeting.

❑ Before you leave, agree on the time, location and agenda for the next meeting and, what, if any, actions need to be taken before that meeting.

Don't be discouraged if the first few meetings don't go as smoothly as you'd hoped. This is a new process. Stick with it and, over time, your family will find a style and format for the meetings that is comfortable and works for everyone.

STEP #3: Get Support

If your parent is in the early stages of the disease, your parent may require little, if any, assistance or care. Other than occasionally repeating a story or misplacing their keys, your parent may have little (or no) behaviors apparent to anyone other than you and your immediate family. Since your parent is probably still capable of taking care of their own needs, their home and most aspects of their life, balancing your parent's needs with the needs of your family, house, life and career may seem effortless. Therefore, getting support may be the last thing on your mind — or you may think you have all the time in the world to get the support you'll eventually need.

Remember, Alzheimer's is a progressive disease so it's not a matter of *if* — but *when* — your parent and your circumstances will change. Sometimes, the changes occur very slowly; other times they come at you quicker than you ever thought humanly possible. If the changes come quickly, you can be caught off-guard and unprepared. You may not have the time or energy to put together a support team or system that truly works for your parent, your family and you.

Find a Support Group

"I can tell you, first and foremost, the top thing someone should do is contact their local Alzheimer's Association chapter. The chapters offer training and education to understand Alzheimer's disease and how to best help the person suffering from it. Many caregivers are overwhelmed by the daunting task of caring for a loved one with Alzheimer's disease. The local chapter of the Alzheimer's Association is there to offer support and guidance."
— Jeffrey A. Asher, Esq., a Trusts & Estates and Elder Law attorney in New York, Trustee of the Alzheimer's Association, NYC Chapter, and former Alzheimer's caregiver.

Caregivers unanimously agree that being involved in an Alzheimer's support group is valuable and necessary for every caregiver. They also say it's important to get involved with a support group as soon after your parent's diagnosis as possible.

Some caregivers, like me, are resistant to the idea of a support group. After a long day of caring for my mom, going to a support group felt like one more thing to do. I also didn't feel comfortable with the idea of sitting in a room full of strangers and sharing intimate details about my mother, myself or our family. But I had a very good friend who kept inviting me to go so, for her, I finally went.

What I found at that first meeting were other people just like me — doing the same thing I was doing and having many of the same struggles and concerns. I also found a place where I didn't feel so alone. I found people who were doing what I was doing, knew what I was going through, and could offer advice based on first-hand experience. I found people who got "it" and got me. I found the Alzheimer's caregivers support group to be a place that:

- Decreased my feelings of isolation.
- Empowered me to be a more confident, capable and loving caregiver.
- Provided me with information on resources available to my mother and our family.
- Gave me an outlet for my emotions and provided much-needed support.

Take the time to find an Alzheimer's support group. Get the
support and information you need. Find people who will get "it"
and get you.

Online Support Groups

Some caregivers, unable to find an Alzheimer's caregivers support
group in their area that fits their needs or their schedule, find support through online support groups and blogs.

Online support groups are available 24/7 which means you
can reach out to them any day, every day, and at a time that is
convenient for you. Caregivers say there was almost always
someone who could relate to what they were going through and
who offered support, advice or suggestions to help them get
through a difficult time with their parent. Even if you're part of a
local support group, you may want to consider an online community for additional support.

The Alzheimer's Association is a good place to begin your
search. You'll find other suggestions in the *Resource* section of
this book.

- Set up a support system. Get hooked in with people who have
  been in your shoes, understand where you're at, can give you
  tips to get through this, or simply be an ear to listen to your
  frustration. So many times, when I was at my wits end, I would
  vent to my friends but all it did was drive them away because
  they didn't understand. Had I not found a group who had been
  on the same journey, I know the journey through Alzheimer's
  would have been much more difficult for me. The tips other
  members of the support system had, through brain storming or
  trial and error, helped us keep Mom at home. — *Chris*

- I attended an Alzheimer's support group meeting and got great
  clarity immediately. We weren't alone! Other families had been
  down this road before! At my first meeting I met a lady whose
  mother had Alzheimer's for many years. I was very fortunate

because she became my mentor and was there for me to lean on.
I also learned that every case is different and that no one else's
story applied to our circumstances because we would have our
own unique story. I immediately called my siblings and encouraged
them to get to a local Alzheimer's support group meeting. — *Dan*

- This is not an easy journey you're on. Be willing to ask for, and accept, help along the way. — *Frank*

- Seek any and all help you can with family, friends, etc. for you and your parent. No one can do this alone. It's simply not possible. — *Gayle*

- Surround yourself with a strong support system of friends and family members. — *Laura*

- Connect with folks farther down the caregiving path who can support you in the days ahead. — *Shelly*

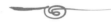

STEP #4: Get Your Legal and Financial Affairs in Order

Paying for your parent's care can cause untold financial and emotional stress on individuals and families — much of which can be
eased by proper advance planning.

Getting your legal and financial affairs in order is a process
that should begin as soon after your parent's diagnosis as possible. Delaying or avoiding this process could have serious implica-
tions for your parent, your family, any existing assets and — most
important — could dictate the level of care you are able to provide for your parent in the months and years to come.

If your parent is still able to participate in this process it may
simplify the process. Having your parent express their wishes can
take some of the guesswork out of this process. Your parent can
also help gather together any legal and financial documents they
already have in place.

If your parent isn't able to participate, you and/or other family members need to locate and assemble the following:

- ❑ Wills, Trusts or Living Trusts.
- ❑ Durable Legal/Medical Power of Attorney.
- ❑ Advance directives for health care (Living will, Do-Not-Resuscitate order, etc.).
- ❑ Deeds, mortgages and any documents relating to real or personal property.
- ❑ Bank and brokerage accounts.
- ❑ Stock and bond certificates.
- ❑ Insurance policies (including Medicare, Medigap, disability, long-term care and life insurance).
- ❑ Any and all other information regarding income or investments including: Social Security, pension or other retirement plans (including individual retirement accounts (IRAs), employee-funded pension plans such as a 401(k), 403(b) and Keough), income from a trust fund or rental properties.
- ❑ Other personal assets (jewelry, artwork, etc.).

Once you have all the documents and information together, consider meeting with an elder care attorney or other trusted legal/financial expert. They will review all existing documents and advise whether they are still applicable considering your parent's and your family's current — and future — circumstances. They can also determine if there are other documents your parent (or family) needs based on finances and your short- and long-term caregiving goals. If there is a chance your parent may one day move to another state or country to be cared for, your advisor can tell you if separate documents need to be prepared since laws can vary between locations.

If you don't have, or know, an elder care attorney or legal/financial advisor, ask others. If you can't afford to pay for these services, check with your state bar association, Legal Aid or Agency on Aging as they, and other community or local agencies, sometimes have low- or no-cost legal services available. Many state and government agencies have sample documents available for download on their websites. See the *Resource* section of this book for additional contact information.

Make copies of legal and other important documents and papers and put them in a safe place. Tell a trusted family member, friend or attorney where they are located. Review the documents regularly to see if changes need to be made as your parent's needs — or family circumstances — change.

Take the time and do what needs to be done *now* to ensure you're able to consistently provide your parent with the level of care they want and deserve.

CAREGIVERS SUGGEST KEEPING THE FOLLOWING INFORMATION UPDATED AND HANDY:

- Your parent's full legal name, their date (and place) of birth and their Social Security number.

- Your parent's education or military records.

- A copy of your parent's most recent income tax return.

- Your parent's employment information, if applicable, including name of their employer and dates of employment.

- Information on your parent's bank accounts, insurance policies, deeds, credit cards and charge accounts.

Organize Your Finances

Individuals with Alzheimer's disease are the highest consumers of long-term care, Medicaid and Medicare, and hospital care. According to the Alzheimer's Association, "People with Alzheimer's disease and other dementias have more than three times as many hospital stays as other older people."[1]

Since many individuals with Alzheimer's often have other medical conditions (diabetes, heart conditions, etc.), it can raise their healthcare costs even further.

Many families mistakenly believe Medicare, and other government programs, will pay for their parent's long-term care. However, the Alzheimer's Association reports that "Although Medicare covers most hospital and other health care services for older people with Alzheimer's and other dementias, individuals and their families still incur high out-of-pocket expenditures for Medicare premiums, deductibles, and co-payments and other health care costs that are not covered by Medicare."[2]

The truth is many families — and individual family members — often end up paying out of their own pocket for some, if not all, of their parent's health care and living expenses, including:

- Housing, food and personal care (either at home or in an assisted living or other facility).
- Ongoing medical treatment and diagnosis.
- Prescription drugs.
- Adult day services.
- In-home or residential care services.
- Hospice or palliative care.

Finances are a constant, recurring concern for most caregivers. Many say even after they thought they had enough money to cover the cost of their parent's care, expenses kept mounting and they remained concerned about being able to pay for their parent's care.

To meet the financial obligations for your parent's care, caregivers suggest you begin where you're at and develop a plan.

Begin Where You're At

Begin by looking at your parent's current financial status including employment income (if they are still working), savings, stocks, bonds, real estate, Social Security, retirement or pension plans, rental income and personal property (such as artwork or jewelry). Review any long-term or healthcare insurance your parent has, either privately or through their employment. Know in advance what the policy covers so you understand what expenses will be your parent's (or your) responsibility to pay for.

If your parent will continue living on their own for a period of time, determine their living expenses by looking at their checkbook and monthly bills. Consider implementing an automatic bill-paying system to ensure your parent's bills are paid on time or by designating a family member to oversee payment of your parent's bills.

Develop a Plan

Even if your parent is living independently, in time they will need the care and oversight of others. There are a number of options as to how to provide ongoing care for your parent. We will discuss care options in more detail in the next chapter but, for now, your family should discuss what individual family members can contribute towards your parent's care either in the form of unpaid care, resources or money. That, along with your parent's resources, will give you an idea of what additional resources you may need in order to provide for your parent's care.

A financial planner, elder care attorney or other professional can also advise you on how to protect as much of your parent's (or family's) existing income and assets as possible so they can be used for your parent's current and ongoing care.

- There are things I wish someone had told me and which I'd like to pass along to other sons and daughters. First, once your parent is diagnosed, begin financial planning. There is a good chance your parent can contribute to important decisions but, even if they can't, the discussion and planning should begin immediately. A durable power of attorney must be named, a will must be created, and a lawyer procured to create these documents. A health care proxy should also be named. This is a very powerful role because, ultimately, decisions for end-of-life care and nursing home admittance rest on this person's shoulder. Your lawyer should also be able to advise you on the Medicare process, etc. Providing care for an Alzheimer's patient is extremely expensive, and chances are, for most people, the patient will run out of money. A family must figure out and communicate what each one is able to contribute financially, if anything, and be advised about the consequences of using the patient's money for expenses not considered appropriate by Medicare. In some instances, a trust should be considered. It is much better off to get this planning out of the way. — *Allyson*

- Pray — then get your financial affairs in order! If your parent is still taking care of their own banking, make sure it is supervised. Otherwise critical mistakes can be made that could be financially devastating. Alzheimer's is a very expensive, time-consuming and emotionally exhausting disease. The last thing your family needs to worry about is how to take care of your parent should assets and bank accounts become inaccessible or mismanaged by your parent. Financial decisions and changes should be made early on while your parent is still capable of making those decisions. Otherwise, the family might not only bear the entire cost of caring for their parent, but also fight to gain access to funds which could be used for caring for their loved one. — *Chris*

- Get organized — now! Begin going through paperwork and get their affairs and paperwork in order. — *David*

- For the sake of everyone involved, make sure anyone with Alzheimer's is not named as the Executor of their spouse's (or anyone else's) estate. — *Jaye*

- Make sure, in addition to knowing where everything is, that you also know the wishes of your parent. It's hard to do, but sensible and necessary. — *Judy*

- Secure a Durable Power of Attorney for health care as well as a Power of Attorney to avoid future legal complications. Consult an attorney experienced in elder law to update Will(s) and explore divestment and/or transfer of assets while your parent is competent. This is important because a person is considered competent until they are legally deemed incompetent — an expensive process which, in my judgment, families should avoid, if at all possible. — *Kitty*

Chapter

4

The Caregiver's Journey

The journey of a caregiver is filled with difficult decisions and multiple demands. In this chapter, we will look at three major demands every Alzheimer's caregiver faces: caring for your parent, caring for the caregiver, and caring for yourself.

PART ONE: Caring For Your Parent

Who Will Care For Mama?

The majority of Alzheimer's caregivers are family members and, oftentimes, several generations of a family. Spouses are often the primary caregiver, followed by a daughter or daughter-in-law. Sons and other family members, including grandchildren, may also provide care.

Deciding who can — or will — care for your parent can be the easiest (or most difficult) decision your family will face. Initially, your family should consider:

- Your parent.
- Your family.
- Your finances.

Consider Your Parent

Begin by considering your parent's current and future mental and physical health and needs. Is your parent still able to cook, clean and care for themselves? If so, perhaps they can continue living independently with oversight and assistance from your family or others. Keep in mind that, even if your parent can live independently, in time, that will change. Eventually, they will need assistance so it may be wise for your family to discuss and have a plan in place before that time comes.

If your parent already needs help with daily tasks, your family needs to decide who will provide that assistance — both now and in the future. There are a number of options — from moving your parent into your home to moving them into a facility and everything in between.

Finally, consider your parent's wishes. Are they still able to provide input — or have they ever expressed their thoughts — on how they would like to be taken care of both now and in the days ahead? While your parent may ask you — or you may want — to promise you'll never place them in a facility, try not to do so. You don't know what the future holds for anyone. Instead, promise your parent you will always make sure they are loved and cared for.

Consider Your Family

Next, consider your family. Consider each family member's health, geographical location and availability. For many families, the spouse (your other parent) is the primary caregiver but is that realistic — both now and in the long term? Are other family members physically, mentally and financially able and willing to take on the role of primary (or back-up) caregiver for your parent?

Even the best care plan will, over time, evolve and change. Your parent's needs will increase or family members' circumstances may shift. Your brother may relocate for his job or your sister may face her own health issues. It's important you — and your family — remain flexible and maintain open lines of communication to address changes as (or before) they happen. It's also imperative for every family member to be open, honest and realistic about how much and what they are willing to give — both now and in the future.

- A family discussion should include what kind of care each person can provide (depending upon their location and other commitments). Not all siblings can, or will, help equally. That is a fact. If nobody wants to — or can — step into the role of primary caregiver, discuss care options. If your parent is able to be a part of this discussion, learning about their wishes will help everyone make decisions further down the line. How comfortable will the patient be with in-home caregivers, or in a facility or nursing home? Don't promise to never place them in a nursing home because, sometimes, it's a promise you can't keep. Consider meeting with a care consultant or other professional trained to help you navigate the road ahead. Make sure you trust the medical personnel on your team and that they are advocates for your parent's care. Make sure the lines of communication remain open and non-confrontational. The stress associated with caring for a patient with Alzheimer's will challenge even the strongest family. — *Allyson*

- It's important to drop all expectations of what other people (siblings, spouse, etc.) should do. Expecting and not getting help from those you love makes things a lot worse. All you can really control is what you do. — *Betsy*

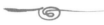

Consider Finances

For many families, a critical — and sometimes the deciding — factor for care options is what their parent, and family, can afford both now and in the future. As we discussed in Chapter Three, with proper planning and assistance it is possible to provide your parent with the type — and level — of care your parent (and you) want.

Just as there are many options as to how your parent will be cared for, there are a number of avenues, options and resources to meet the cost of that care. These include:

❑ Family income and assets: You, and your family members, may want to consider your own assets and income to see what, if any, amount you can contribute towards your parent's care — both now and in the future. Also look into any possible work-related benefits — from paid time off to medical coverage or diagnostic testing for your parent.

❑ Healthcare coverage (private policy, group health plan provided by their employer, or retiree health coverage): If your parent has recently left their employment, they may also qualify for COBRA group coverage.

❑ Medicare, Medicaid or Medigap.

❑ Disability insurance (private policy or through an employer).

❑ Private healthcare or long-term care insurance.

❑ Life insurance.

❑ State Health Insurance Assistance Program (SHIP).

❑ National Family Caregiver Support Program (NFCSP).

❑ Partnership for Prescription Assistance (PPA).

❑ Social Security Disability Income (SSDI).

❑ Veterans' benefits.

Many communities offer low-cost or free programs and services including adult day care and/or respite care, meal delivery programs, support groups, transportation, and hospice or palliative care. Many religious and community organizations have help available even to non-members.

Caregivers should also ask an accountant or tax expert about possible tax deductions and credits, including the Household and Dependent Care Credit, for the caregiver.

See the *Resource* section of this book for contact information.

The Family as Caregiver

Some families approach caregiving as a team with individual family members taking on tasks that match their strengths or abilities. Team caregiving requires a lot of advance planning as well as open, and continuous, communication between family members. It can also be a wonderful experience for the entire family.

As things changed, we continued to meet and make adjustments and divide up responsibilities based on availability, skills and resources. For the most part, my sister (who lived closest to Mom and Dad) became our "point person." She helped care for Dad and was the one who kept her finger on the pulse of what was happening so she could relay that information to the rest of us. Having one point person allowed all of us to hear the same information and avoided any miscommunication or misinterpretation between family members.

Others who lived at a distance helped out by handling our parents' finances and paperwork. We also called on a regular basis to talk to Dad or to check in on Mom and my sister. When it seemed the demands on Mom or my sister were beginning to overwhelm them, one of us would come and stay to give them a break.

Since my sister had to stop working to help Mom with Dad's care — and since the rest of us were able to continue working — we all decided to contribute to a fund that would pay our sister. Initially, my sister felt uncomfortable with this but we explained that the alternative was paying someone outside the family to help care for Dad. I think, in the end, she was grateful she was able to continue caring for Dad — and to remain financially solvent in the process. — **Frank**

♡

My father was 96 when he was diagnosed with Alzheimer's. My mother was 72 and in great health. I was 36 and the second youngest of seven children.

This was our family's first experience with Alzheimer's so I scoured the Internet to find out everything and anything I could about the disease. I think what I feared the most was that Dad would run away or get into someone's car and take off. Gratefully, neither ever happened.

We worked together as a family. My mother, my husband, my children and I took care of my father on a daily basis. My brothers and sisters are scattered throughout the country. Some were able to help more than others but we all talked and made decisions as a family regarding my father's care. We were all very supportive and talked to Mom constantly.

Even though Mom was in great health, I still worried about her. I was worried she might have a nervous breakdown or hurt herself while trying to bathe him or care for him.

At one point, Dad realized he forgot my name. He looked at me and said, "Honey, I forgot your name." I just smiled and said, "Daddy, you've been calling me 'Honey' forever." He smiled, obviously relieved.

He was always such a clean, proper and dignified man. I'm grateful he didn't know what was happening to him.

Dad ended up dying from a massive stroke two years after he was diagnosed with Alzheimer's. During the two years we cared for him, I believe we did a lot of things right in caring for him. There is honestly nothing I wish we had done differently. We kept him home and he was very comfortable. We laughed, and cried, together and loved him unconditionally. We worked together and through it all we became a much closer family. — **Lois**

♡

My parents, though very different, always complemented one another and had an unusually happy marriage. My father was the one to identify problems, plan a solution and reach out for resources. Now that he is intellectually paralyzed by Alzheimer's, he can no longer do those things and Mom, for her own painful reasons, refuses to pick up the reins. Dad is the only person in whom Mom has ever confided so she isn't coping terribly well with his decline. Denial is her sole means of handling problems so most attempts to address any problems directly are met with non-verbalized hostility — which she bottles up as best she can.

I am my parents' youngest child and only daughter. I have three brothers and we all live very far from my par-

ents. Like any family, we have our tensions, but there are no deeply-rooted conflicts among us. There are, however, varied connections which reflect and, to a great extent, determine our engagement with our parents' suffering.

As my father's condition worsens, my mother's anger with me (and him) gets more and more unbearable. I think, for my mother, in some ways I have come to symbolize the embodiment of the disease itself. My father's illness enrages her; my father enrages her; I enrage her.

*Mom is still struggling through her days trying to care for my dad, enduring her terrible loss in silence and solitude. However, the quasi-good news is that we seem to be joining together a little bit now. While one of my brothers still has his head stuck in the sand trap at his golf club, the rest of us are finding our sea legs — which is a good thing since the waters are starting to get a lot rougher. We seem to be dividing up tasks to some extent and I feel lucky the workload is being shared more than in many families. If we manage not to hate each other by the end of this, it will be a testament to my parents' kindness and decency. We had a good life as children, and we owe them good teamwork in their darkest hour. — **Pam***

♡

My dad has Alzheimer's. My mom is his caregiver although we all take time to help. My husband and I spend every Friday with Dad. My brothers and their wives take Dad to and from an Alzheimer's program two days a week so Mom doesn't have to. We are all closeby and visit regularly. It is my fervent hope (and I tell Mom this regularly) that if she needs us, she'll let us know.
*— **Wanda***

Long-Distance Caregiving

Typically, long-distance caregivers live an hour, or more, from their parent. In some instances, they are the primary caregiver for their parent. Other times, they provide back-up support to the primary caregiver. At the outset, a long-distance caregiver's responsibilities may include calling their parent several times throughout the day to check on them or handling their finances. However, as the disease progresses, it may mean arranging for their parent's in-home care or providing occasional respite care to the primary caregiver.

If you are a long-distance caregiver, it's important when you visit or talk with your parent to remain observant and mindful of:

- ❑ **Your parent's appearance:** Is your parent clean and well-groomed? Does it look as though they are bathing regularly? Or are they, or their clothes, dirty and unkempt?

- ❑ **Your parent's home and surroundings:** What is the condition of their home (both inside and out)? Is mail piled up or unopened? Check their refrigerator to see what they are eating and if the food is spoiled. Does it look as though the house is being maintained?

- ❑ **What your parent says and does:** Are they getting increasingly confused or agitated? In telephone conversations, do they talk about being unable to find things in their home? Do you notice that it is taking them longer to get home from the grocery store? If so, it could be an indication that they are having difficulty finding their way home and are getting lost.

- ❑ **What others say:** When you visit your parent, talk with neighbors and friends to get an outsider's perspective on how your parent is doing. Try to schedule your parent's doctor's appointments so you can go along and get a professional opinion on your parent's overall physical and mental health and well-being.

Make sure you have information on (or copies of) your parent's health, financial and legal records. This is particularly important if there is an emergency — or if the primary caregiver has an emergency — and you have to come in on short notice. It will lessen your learning curve and allow you to be an effective caregiver for your parent.

Long-distance caregivers, while not dealing with the hands-on responsibilities of caregiving, still deal with the emotions and concerns of other caregivers. They worry and are anxious. They often experience bouts of guilt or remorse since they aren't closer or physically present for their parent. Long-distance caregivers may also feel they aren't spending enough time with their parent or doing enough to help.

If you are a long-distance caregiver, find a support group in your community or online where you can talk to others who are providing long-distance care for their parent. It may be helpful to know you aren't alone.

Providing Care At Home

Many families, at least initially, care for their parent at home. Caring for your parent at home means you (and any other caregivers) are responsible for dressing, bathing, meals, medication, toileting, and social activities. You are responsible for everything. If you decide to care for your parent at home, it will mean major changes to your life — and your home.

At first, changes may be something as simple as making sure items are kept in the same place or labeling drawers so your parent can find things easily. However, as the disease progresses, you'll need to make additional — and sometimes major — modifications to your home to keep your parent safe, to help them remain independent as long as possible, and to reduce difficult behaviors, such as wandering.

We will discuss modifications to your home and ensuring your parent's safety in greater detail in Chapter Five but, for now, consider the following:

- ❑ Keep furnished areas simple and uncomplicated.
- ❑ Minimize clutter.
- ❑ Avoid re-arranging furniture or moving items in the home.
- ❑ Keep items in the same place to serve as a visual cue for your parent to acclimate themselves and remember where they are.
- ❑ Adjust the lighting — inside and outside the home — depending upon the time of day and activity.

❑ During mealtime, lowering the lights may keep your parent calm and improve their eating habits.

❑ At night, adjust lights to reduce or eliminate shadows and reduce the possibility of hallucinations.

Think about, and discuss with other family members, how moving your parent into your home will impact your life and your family. Be honest with yourself — and your family — about whether you are prepared for such an undertaking. It is better to be honest at the outset and come up with an alternative plan than to go forward and move your parent into your home — or you move into theirs — only to find you, or your parent, is unhappy, resentful, or unsafe.

Some caregivers say moving their parent into their home seemed like an ideal situation but, looking back, there are things they wish they'd considered. Caregivers suggest, in advance of any move, you consider:

❑ Your ability to meet your parent's continuing — and constantly changing — needs.

❑ How much of a transition it will be, not just for you and your family, but for your parent.

❑ How far you will have to travel for medical, dental or other services for your parent.

❑ What modifications you will have to make to your home — and life — to ensure your parent's comfort and safety.

❑ How the move will impact any young children or teenagers at home.

❑ How it will impact you, your life and your personal freedoms.

❑ How it will impact your ability to get together or socialize with others both in, and away from, your home.

❑ How it will impact your family's finances, both now and in the future (especially if you have to stop working to care for your parent).

❑ How it will feel to have someone be dependent on you every second of every day.

❑ How you will continue to cope, day in and day out, with an increasingly difficult situation.

❑ How having your parent living with you could mean becoming a "prisoner" in your own home.

❑ What respite and support services are available in your family and community.

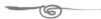

My mother was diagnosed with Alzheimer's at the age of 76. Mom had been widowed twice and I believe my stepfather's death was the beginning of Mom's confusion.

My sister moved in with Mom after my stepfather's death to help her through the changes. She kept telling me she thought Mom was slipping mentally but I didn't see it. Then we all went on a trip together and, when I finally spent more than a weekend with my mother, I realized what my sister was talking about.

My sister lived with my mother for over ten years but then my sister died suddenly of heart failure. Eight months later, my brother died from cancer. With both of my siblings gone, the responsibility of caring for Mom full-time was mine. I knew she wasn't happy at the assisted living home where she'd been for over a year and I wasn't happy driving three hours every weekend to visit her.

My husband, Carl, and I did a lot of talking, soul searching and praying, and finally decided to move Mom in with us. Carl and I have been married for almost 30 years. He is my husband and my best friend and, without his support and help taking care of Mom, I don't know if I would have been able to do this.

*There has definitely been a learning curve for me. I thought I knew what we were getting ourselves into but there is no way to be totally ready to care for a parent with Alzheimer's. You just have to do it one day at a time. I also know this is something I need to do for me as much as for Mom. — **Bonnie***

I was married and living in North Carolina when Mama was first diagnosed. She was living in Chicago near one of my sisters.

I am the youngest of four girls and together, my sisters and I bought Mama a condominium so she could keep her independence. Another sister and I sent money and we all talked regularly and made decisions together about Mama's care.

On one of my visits to Chicago, Mama was underweight and looked terrible. I talked with my sisters and told them I was thinking of quitting my job to care for her. They agreed. Since I was fortunate to be in a financial position to quit my job, I brought Mama to live with me and began caring for her full-time.

Mama gained weight and, for a while, was doing well. Then, slowly, she started getting worse, both physically and mentally. She would fall out of bed and I couldn't pick her up. At the time, my husband was working a lot and wasn't home to help me. I talked with my sisters and we briefly considered putting Mama into a nursing home. Gratefully, we never did.

*Mama knew something was wrong. She also knew she was powerless over the disease and there was nothing she could do to keep her memory. Even though it was very stressful, I'm never sorry I took care of her. I'm grateful I was able to share Mama's last years with her — that I was able to do her hair, take her to the beach and out to eat, put make-up on her, bathe her and love her so much. — **Grace***

I hated that my father-in-law, whom I loved very much, had Alzheimer's. Even though it was really hard at times, I'm grateful I was able to move into his home and take care of him. I wanted him to have as normal a life as possible. It was the least I could do to repay him for all the kindness and love he gave to me after I married his son and was privileged to become a part of their family. And when we were in the final stages with Dad, I was glad I was there to care for him, bathe him, and keep him comfortable. — **Marie**

For some caregivers, their experience of caring for their parent is very different than the caregivers above. Even though a difficult relationship, long-standing problems or a lifetime of resentments may still exist between them and their parent, some caregivers still attempt to care for their parent. For many, the hope is that it will finally bring some healing to their relationship with their parent. Sometimes that happens. For others, as in the case of the following caregiver, it soon became obvious that it was better for everyone to have someone else care for their parent.

One year after my stepfather died, his family told us my mother had dementia. The fact that our family didn't know about my mother's condition wasn't completely his (or my mother's) fault. I knew my mother's memory had been failing but I was uninformed about Alzheimer's.

My mother and I never had a good relationship. Nonetheless, following her hip replacement surgery, I invited her to come live with me. I really believed it could work.

I am hard-pressed to express the depth of the agony I experienced. It was completely unexpected. I had no one to help me and soon learned that caring for someone with Alzheimer's is not something you can do without a lot of help. Money, too, became an issue. But the isolation and financial strain were nothing compared to the anguish I felt at having this vindictive, mean-spirited woman in my home.

My mother treated me with contempt. People would tell me it was "the disease, not her" but I felt the disease was only allowing more of the "real her" to come out. Here I was, a middle-aged woman, feeling the same emotional and psychological torment I endured my entire childhood. All the literature for caregivers reminds us to take care of our own health first. I am forever grateful to my friend who reminded me that included not just my physical but my mental health.

When I told that same friend I was thinking of moving my mother into an assisted living facility at the end of the summer, his first words to me were, "Why wait?" Those words gave me the strength to find a place and, rather quickly, I moved her.

I admit I had no difficulty putting my mother into a facility. Most days, I don't worry about her or whether I did the right thing. Most days, I'm busy with my own life. If that sounds selfish, so be it. I fail to see the point in both of us stewing in a broth of discontent and resentment.

This isn't to say I haven't felt guilty but when I read the posts from caregivers on the online Alzheimer's forums, I can't relate to their declarations of love and endless sacrifice. This hasn't been my experience with my mother so it's outside my realm of understanding.

I'm writing this because I know there are other people like me. People who have (or had) a difficult relationship with their parent, people who feel more hate than love towards their parent. I also need those who never had this kind of relationship to understand and not judge us.

I'm still responsible for my mother's paperwork. I'm blessed that my only surviving brother (there were once four of us) and my aunt help me.

*A silence has been broken in our family and we are healing a little at a time. I still have a lot of bitterness but slowly optimism is beginning to bloom once again — an optimism that reminds me I am a person who deserves to be treated with dignity. My mother wasn't the only person to be considered in this situation. — **Joy***

Meeting Your Parent's Ongoing Care Needs

As the disease progresses, you may struggle to meet your parent's ever-changing and ever-increasing needs. If you don't get a break or respite from your duties as a caregiver, it can result in caregiver burnout and could ultimately impact your health.

Respite care can include any, or all, of the following:

- Companion services (supervision or visitation with your parent).
- Personal care services (assistance with hygiene, bathing, etc.).
- Skilled care services (assisting with your parent's medical needs including monitoring and dispensing medication).
- Homemaker services (assistance with meal preparation, shopping and housekeeping).

Respite care provides you with a much-needed break while also ensuring your parent receives the care or attention they require.

Some families get respite care through a support network of family, friends, neighbors, church members and others. Some hire live-in help while others turn to other forms of respite care, such as adult day programs, volunteer care or paid respite care.

Adult day centers and programs are typically run by a highly-trained staff. These centers provide supervision for your parent along with activities that encourage your parent's independence and cognitive abilities. Adult day centers may be a viable option if you need supervision for your parent while you work or run errands since most programs are available for either a few hours or the whole day. Many caregivers say the extra stimulation and social opportunities the adult day center provides results in decreased wandering, restlessness and sleeping difficulties for their parent. Many adult care centers also provide a meal or snack during the day.

Some caregivers receive unpaid, or volunteer, respite care in their home through a relative, neighbor, or friend. Community and religious organizations often have a "Friendly Visitor Program" which provides volunteers who can provide basic respite care even if you aren't a member or affiliated with the organization.

Another option is short-term respite care for your parent through a nursing home, hospital or residential home. This can be difficult to arrange since it requires a room being available for your parent at a specific time. However, some care facilities and hospitals reserve a number of rooms for short-term care or, if you can be flexible, you may be able to work your respite around availability at the facility.

If financial concerns are holding you back from asking for or receiving help, look and see what is available in your area. Ask members of your local Alzheimer's support group for referrals or advice. Contact your local Agency on Aging (or other local or community agencies) to see if there are local, state or federal programs that might offer either respite programs or financial assistance. Review your parent's insurance policy to see if they have coverage for respite care.

You might also consider the age-old system of bartering. Perhaps someone in your family who isn't a full-time caregiver can provide a service to someone in exchange for that person providing you with a much-needed break. Maybe your brother could fix the neighbor's fence or your son or daughter could rake a friend's leaves in exchange for your neighbor or friend staying with your parent for an hour, or an afternoon.

Many individuals diagnosed with Alzheimer's receive care at home from family and friends. However, since providing continuing care for your parent is both challenging and stressful, it's important the caregiver understands and accepts their personal limitations. It's also important to find resources to support the caregiver and be prepared to ask for, and accept, help.

One form of support is home health care. There are two main types of home health care: medical and non-medical.

Medical home health care means there is a "skilled need". It may be a nurse or other medical professional coming into the home to provide physical therapy, wound care or other service to your parent. Medicare and HMOs may cover the cost of this type of homecare for a specific period of time depending upon your circumstances.

Non-medical home care addresses the everyday needs of an individual: companionship, light housekeeping, bathing, dressing or feeding. These services are typically provided by sources other than medical professionals, such as a community-based or private business or organization, or through a network of friends, family or other caregivers.

There are a number of ways to cover the cost of home health care. Your private insurance may cover the cost or Medicaid waiver programs often provide financial assistance for care for individuals who qualify for nursing home care but prefer to remain at home. For veterans, there are programs, such as the Aid and Attendance Program, which can support a family's effort to keep a loved one at home as long as possible.

I have compiled a list of questions on my website (see *Resource* section of this book) to further assist you in finding home health care that is right for you and your parent.

Diane Carbo, RN has over 35 years of experience as a registered nurse and as an advocate for older adults and their families.

Making the Move to a Care Facility

In the later stages of the disease, your parent will require twenty-four hour care. As much as caregivers and their family want to continue caring for their parent at home, there often comes a time when they are no longer able to provide the level or type of care their parent needs. At that point, families often decide to move their parent into a residential care facility.

This can be an extremely difficult, heart-wrenching decision for many caregivers and their family. Some resist making the move, even though their own health is compromised, because they feel such a move means they have in some way given up, failed or abandoned their parent. Even when it is apparent that a move to a care facility is the right (and loving) decision for your parent, caregivers often experience a number of emotions including grief, sadness and guilt.

As one of our caregivers, pointed out, the deciding when, where, or if your parent should be moved is very personal. No one can, or should, tell you if this is the right choice for your parent or your family.

My advice to anyone who wants to keep their parent at home is to search your heart long and hard. This is a tough road and it will wear you out, physically and mentally. If you decide to keep your parent at home, know that you can't do it alone. And often, unless there's a hefty bank *account, there aren't enough resources. Don't let anyone make you feel guilty if you have to move your parent into a care facility. Every situation is different. — **Gayle***

Caregivers also say there are a number of factors to consider when making the decision, including:

❑ Are you able to provide constant — and consistent — care for your parent?

❑ Does your parent require more help than you, your family, or your extended care network is able to provide?

❑ Has your parent become physically abusive or combatant?

❑ Do you ever worry about your parent's — or your own — safety?

❑ Are you, or another caregiver, struggling or suffering (physically, emotionally, or mentally) to care for your parent?

❑ Are you, or another caregiver, jeopardizing your own physical or mental health by caring for your parent?

❑ Are you, or any other caregiver, having difficulty balancing your caregiving responsibilities with the responsibilities of your family, home or work?

❑ Is providing care for your parent causing a financial hardship on you or your family?

If you answered "Yes" to any of the above, it may be time to consider other care options, including the possibility of moving your parent to a care facility.

Choosing the Right Facility

Even if you're not currently considering moving your parent, it's wise to plan for the *possibility* of a move. Caregivers recommend researching what facilities and care options exist near your parent (or the primary caregiver) well in advance of any *actual* move. Visit every facility to determine if it meets the needs of your parent and your family.

Be aware that you may experience a range of emotions — from sadness to relief — during your visit. Visiting the facility may also provide you with some clarity as to whether it's the right time — or decision — to move your parent.

Prior to your visit, prepare a list of things to look for along with a list of questions. You may want to know their staff-to-resident ratio or what services or programs they have for an Alzheimer's patient and their family. You might want to know what the meal and food options are for residents or how they handle emergency and non-emergency situations. You might ask to see their most recent inspection report and if they are licensed by the state.

You can tell a lot about a facility simply by watching the people who work and live there. Does the staff interact with, and appear to genuinely care for, the residents? Do they seem interested in getting to know your parent, you and other family members or are they rushed and unapproachable? Do the residents seem comfortable and happy? Do they appear well taken care of? Is the facility warm and inviting? Is it clean? Is it safe?

It's also important to determine the cost so you can begin finding the necessary financial resources.

The bottom line in your choice is: are you confident this is a place where your parent will be well cared for? If so, ask if there is a waiting list, find out the wait time, and consider placing your parent's name on the list. Caregivers say it helped to have their parent's name on the list well in advance of the move so that, when the time came, they didn't lose valuable time (and resources) finding a place for their parent.

Caregivers say knowing a facility met all of the qualifications and criteria set by their family helped relieve some of the emotions associated with moving their parent.

Preparing For the Move

❏ If your parent hasn't been part of the decision-making process, you'll need to consider how you are going to tell them about the move. Plan what you are going to say in advance of the actual conversation — as well as who is going to tell them. If your parent is close to one particular individual it may be wise to allow that person to tell them. Or your family may want to talk to your parent together.

❑ When having the actual discussion, keep it short and simple. Be consistent — and use the same words — in both your explanation and your answers to any questions your parent may have.

❑ Anticipate a reaction from your parent. While not all caregivers say their parents reacted negatively to the news, some said their parents flatly refused to go or got extremely agitated, angry or sad. Honor and acknowledge your parent's feelings.

❑ Some families opt to not tell their parent in advance of the actual move. How your parent has reacted to events in the past — and whether it helped or upset them to know about things in advance — will help you decide what is right for your parent and family.

❑ If possible, complete all paperwork in advance of the move to allow you to be completely present — physically and emotionally — for your parent on the day of the move.

❑ Some facilities allow you to decorate a room in advance of the move. If you can, consider decorating your parent's room in the facility similar to their bedroom at home.

❑ Put together a photo album or collage of family photos — not only for your parent's comfort but also to allow the staff to get to know your parent. This also creates opportunities for the staff to interact and talk with your parent.

❑ Many facilities have a form on which you can list your parent's interests, routine or other personal information. If they don't, consider preparing such a list yourself.

The Day of the Move

❑ Introduce yourself to the staff and, if possible, find out who will be primarily caring for your parent.

❑ Tell the staff any "inside information" that might be helpful in caring for your parent. If your parent has pet names for things, let them know. If your family is calling the facility your parent's "new apartment" let the staff know. Tell the staff anything that will help them assist your parent to adjust both before, during and after the move.

❑ Bring along some of your parent's favorite personal items — pictures, blankets, books, or even a chair or other piece of furniture — to help personalize your parent's space and make them feel more comfortable and at home.

❑ Remain upbeat and positive. Smile. If you think you're going to be sad or cry, you may want to ask another family member or friend to do the actual move.

❑ Devote the entire day to the move. While it may not physically take you all day to move, allow your parent — and yourself — time to adjust. Some facilities allow you to stay with your parent while others prefer you leave to allow your parent time to settle into their new surroundings.

❑ If you are having difficulty determining how, or the best time, to leave your parent, ask the staff for assistance. They have had experience with this and may have some helpful, or creative, solutions that will make your departure easier on your parent — and you.

After the Move

❑ If possible, visit your parent within a few days of the move so they don't feel abandoned.

❑ Call or visit as often as possible.

❑ Acknowledge your parent's feelings. They may get agitated, confused or withdrawn when you visit.

❑ Allow your parent time to adjust. You may find your parent thrives in the new environment due to the increased activity and socialization.

❑ Even if your parent adjusts to a facility, be prepared that *you* might have feelings of anger, loss, sadness or guilt after the move. This is extremely normal and is part of the ongoing grieving process of loving and caring for your parent. Allow yourself to feel any and all emotions since it is all part of the healing process — and know you have made a loving decision based on what is best for your parent.

❑ Requests by your parent to "go home" may be their way of expressing a desire to see family or loved ones who have died. It isn't always about returning back to their home as they may no longer remember where "home" is.

❑ Volunteer or keep your family involved in your parent's daily and group activities. You might consider bringing the family pet to visit or an activity that you and your parent always enjoyed doing together.

❑ Get to know the staff, including any new staff members, and address them by name.

❑ Don't forget to praise and thank the staff. A simple and sincere "thank you" goes a long way.

❑ Maintain open communication and build a relationship with the staff and, in particular, your parent's caregivers. As much as possible, have the same staff members care for your parent so they can get to know your parent — and vice versa. When you visit, try to connect with those staff members to get updates on how your parent is doing.

❑ Shift changes can be stressful for your parent due to increased noise and activity and new faces coming on the scene. If possible, have a family member there to ease the transition.

❑ Choose your battles wisely. Every residence — and staff member — has good and bad days. It's important to know what issues are worth fighting over and which ones will only make the situation worse.

❑ It may be helpful to have a family member present for baths.

❑ If you begin to question the care your parent is receiving, begin looking at other facilities. Don't settle.

Our initial goal was to allow my husband's mother, Anna, to maintain her independence as long as possible by staying in the home where she had lived for 45 years. Ever since Tom's father died, Anna was living alone on the family farm. She had two sisters and a brother who lived nearby and we lived 100 miles away.

When we visited Anna, we noticed she had very little food in her pantry and that items were misplaced or in strange places around her house. Her doctor (who is a close family friend) also expressed his concerns about her forgetfulness to Tom.

Then, in December 2007, Anna locked herself out of the house. A neighbor came to check on his livestock which he kept at Anna's farm and found her, cold and freezing, on the porch. He helped Anna into the house and called us.

We decided to have Anna come live with us. Three months after she moved in, two doctors agreed she had Alzheimer's and declared her incompetent. She was 77 years old.

During the two years Anna lived with us, Tom and I shared the responsibility of caring for her. I'm a stay-at-home mom with two young children so most of the daytime tasks fell under my supervision. Tom made all the medical-related decisions since he is Anna's healthcare power of attorney and was also very involved in Anna's daily care.

*As the disease progressed, a family decision was made to move Anna into a facility so she could receive constant, professional care. Anna now resides in an Alzheimer's wing at a care facility about 10 miles from our home. — **Alissa***

♡

My mother is the oldest of four sisters. None of her sisters were ever diagnosed with Alzheimer's. Mom is the first. The only.

After my father died, Mom moved into an apartment near my brother but, soon after she moved, my brother was diagnosed with cancer. When he died, my mother became very depressed.

Although Mom was probably having problems before my brother died, we didn't really notice until afterwards. They were small things — like forgetting an ingredient in a recipe or calling and telling me she'd "done the silliest thing today" — but they were now happening more frequently.

Since Mom didn't drive she relied on friends to take her places. Many of those friends began to express their concern also. They said Mom would call and ask for a ride but, when they arrived, Mom would still be in her nightgown and had no memory of ever calling them.

That summer, every time I talked to Mom she didn't sound right. I told my husband if I didn't know any better I'd think my mother had started drinking because she sounded like she was drunk. It came on so suddenly that I knew something was wrong so my husband and I brought Mom to live with us to figure out what was going on.

Before long, we discovered the problem: Mom was forgetting she'd already taken her medication and was taking another dose the same day. She was accidentally overdosing on her medication.

I immediately took charge of Mom's medication and her odd behavior vanished. I then called a family meeting to discuss with my brother and sisters what we should do. My siblings recommended putting Mom in an assisted living facility so Mom and I went to visit a really nice place near my home. The entire time, Mom kept saying "Please don't do this to me." I couldn't do it so we moved to Plan B: we found a ground-level apartment in a senior complex just around the corner from my house.

Mom is still able to dress herself every morning and make her own breakfast. I had my husband shut the gas off to her stove so I don't have to worry about her cooking. She loves having tea and toast in the morning and, since she has a microwave and toaster, she's still able to make her own breakfast.

I start my day by getting my three children fed and

dressed. I drop them off at school and then pick Mom up and take her to an adult day program. At the end of the day, I pick up my kids, then my mom, and we all come back to our house and have dinner together. Afterwards, we talk or watch TV. Since Mom loves to help, I give her small chores like folding laundry or clipping coupons. I give Mom her medication and then, around 8:00 or 8:30 PM, I take her home. I put her clothes out for the next day, and get her settled in bed. She's usually exhausted from her day and is ready to go to sleep.

Lately, I've begun to worry more and more about Mom. Her confusion seems to be getting worse. She'll call me sometimes at 2:00 AM and ask where I am. I tell her I'm home in bed and she'll tell me she's dressed and waiting to go to the adult day center. She has no concept of time. She's also getting really paranoid. She tells me my kids are lost when they're actually in the house. She just doesn't remember.

She wears a LifeAlert bracelet which gives me some relief but it's only effective if Mom remembers to press the button. I worry what would happen if she wandered off in the middle of the night.

I'm lucky. My family is very supportive. My husband and children have been great — and I know this hasn't been easy on them. One of my sisters made me promise that if caring for Mom ever began to affect me, my marriage, or my family life, I would move Mom to an assisted living facility.

Over the winter, Mom got shingles. She was in so much pain and I was trying to be with her and also care for my children. It was impossible for one person to give Mom the amount of care she needed while also caring for three children. It just about did me in.

My sister came up, took one look at me and said, "Karen, I love you, but I think you're making yourself sick. Let's go look at assisted living again."

Right now, we're on a waiting list for an assisted living facility near our home but I don't look forward to moving

*Mom. I'll miss her. I love her. I'm just worried about her. I just want her to be safe and happy. — **Karen B.***

♡

The first time I noticed anything was on New Year's Day 2000. My parents were at my sister's wedding and Dad, who was 82, was slower and not as sharp.

The following Christmas, my parents wanted to come visit me. They lived on Cape Cod and I live in New Jersey and, since they no longer drove long distances, I drove up to get them. On the trip back to New Jersey, I noticed we needed to stop more often than usual so Daddy could use the men's room. I also noticed he was relying on Mom to give him his medication, help him around a "strange" house, and to just be there for him.

The following Thanksgiving, Daddy suffered a stroke and was in a rehab center for over a year. While he was there, he lost a lot of weight, didn't remember things, and said things totally out-of-character. The nurses loved him because he was so sweet and helpful but he also got very sad, angry and frightened while he was there. It was obvious he was also becoming more disoriented. Every time my sisters and I visited him, we would have to tell him who we were, where we lived, and how many children we had. He was forgetting so much and it scared him. He often said he wanted to be with his "Ma and Pa."

After he returned home, Mom tried to take care of him by herself but he started having a series of TIA strokes. At one point, he fell and Mom wasn't able to lift him so, once again, he was hospitalized and, once again, was sent to rehab.

Mom was 81 years old but she still did all the driving, cleaning, shopping and caring for their home and cats. She had been his sole caregiver and you could see it was starting to take its toll on her. My sisters and I finally told Mom what she already knew: that she simply could no longer do it alone and it would be better for both of them if Daddy moved into a facility.

We found a wonderful facility where we could visit at all hours. My sister was even allowed to bring her young son to visit. We brought Daddy gifts, made noise and took him for rides in his wheelchair in the hallway — or outside if the weather was nice. We tried to make Daddy feel that even though he was no longer at home, his family was — and would always be — with him.

This second time in rehab was much tougher because even though we all knew it was where he needed to be we all knew that, this time, my father wouldn't be coming home. — **Roberta**

Our final story is from Allyson. You first met Allyson in Chapter Two when she was still caring for her father in her home. However, over time and during the course of writing this book, things changed for Allyson and her father. Here is the continuation of her journey with her father and Alzheimer's.

I took care of Dad for four years in my home. During that time, his needs were changing constantly so I spent a lot of time thinking, and preparing, for his future care. I researched Alzheimer's residential places and called them to do a phone interview. I recorded their responses to my questions on a spreadsheet and visited the ones that seemed to be the best fit for my dad.

We finally found one we really liked and I had Dad's name placed on a waiting list. Several times, his name came to the top of the list but I wasn't quite ready for him to move out of our home yet.

Following stent surgery Dad didn't gain back the strength in his legs and was having some balance problems. I could see he was at risk for a fall. I was particularly concerned because Dad's bedroom was on the second floor and he had started wandering at night. I was so afraid he would fall down the stairs. His confusion was deepening and he didn't always recognize me any longer.

Dad needed 24/7 care because of the nighttime wander-

ing. I tried various caregivers and agencies over the years but nothing really seemed to work out. There was also no one in my family to back me up because they either lived at a distance or had their own health concerns. I grew increasingly concerned over what might happen should I get sick or become disabled. I also knew, if I waited too long to move Dad, we ran the risk he would have difficulty learning his way around the assisted living facility.

Gratefully, around this time, a spot opened up at the facility, so I began to prepare to move him out of our home.

During the next phase of the move, I was fairly calm and treated it like a Project Manager. I had daily lists of how to move his things to the home without Dad knowing. I was so busy getting the move coordinated — ensuring his room there was like his room in our house and giving the facility information on how to work with him — that I didn't get very emotional at that point.

On the day of the move, my family helped. I didn't feel I could be the one to drop Dad off so my sister and brother-in-law did that part. It actually went really well. They told Dad the Admissions Director was an old high school friend, and she took Dad's arm and showed him around and he loved it! I called later that day and told him we had a medical emergency with my husband's father in England. I called every few days but I didn't see him for two and a half weeks.

The worst part of the move for me was how much I missed Dad. He was such a delight and we had so many rituals that gave him consistency. I just missed his company.

Dad was doing really well and my mind was at peace that he was in the best possible place for him. Everything was fine until he fell and broke his hip.

As prepared as I was for the residential facility, I wasn't prepared at all for the skilled nursing/rehab facility where he is now. I had to make very quick decisions without enough time to think things through. This was further complicated by having to change plans since Dad was now residing in a different state.

The rehab where Dad is doesn't have enough activities for him. While there may be other facilities that would provide him with more activities, I'm not sure I want to move him again at this point. My hope is that he can learn to use the walker and we can move him back to the residential care facility where he was before he fell.

PART TWO: Caring For the Caregiver

The Spouse as Caregiver

For many families, the primary caregiver is the spouse — your other parent. While that may seem like a loving, and logical, choice it can also add one more level of concern for a son or daughter. In a perfect world, the spouse is in extremely good health — both physically and mentally. However, since Alzheimer's strikes individuals in their later years, there is a chance the spouse may be facing their own health concerns. Therefore, having the spouse as the primary caregiver often means a son or daughter now has to be diligent about — and concerned for — the health and welfare of both of their parents.

Studies show caregivers experience high levels of stress, frustration, anxiety, exhaustion and anger which can result in depression, increased use of alcohol or other substances, reduced immune response, and poor physical health.

Many caregivers say, as time passed, they saw the spouse growing more and more exhausted, stressed or depressed. Some families ended up having to place their parent with Alzheimer's in a long-term facility simply because the spouse's health had deteriorated to the point where it was no longer safe or feasible for them to continue to provide care.

Caregivers say to watch and see if the spouse:

❑ Is falling more frequently.

❑ Has unexplained bruising, cuts or scratches.

❑ Has poor eating habits or isn't getting adequate nutrition.

❑ Is neglecting their own personal care and hygiene.

☐ Is having difficulty following doctor's orders or dosage instructions on medication.

☐ Is beginning to have bouts with forgetfulness or memory loss.

If you notice any of the above, it may be an indication that the spouse's health or safety is in jeopardy or that additional help is needed. Even when it is obvious that additional help is needed, many caregivers say the spouse was resistant to ask for, or accept, help. That may be due to a number of factors.

First, some spouses resist sharing caregiving responsibilities with anyone because, after so many years of marriage, they feel they know the person with Alzheimer's better than anyone else and are the only one capable of providing proper and adequate care.

Another reason may be that the spouse doesn't see the need for help. Since the spouse is with your parent most or all of the time, they may not see the subtle (and not so subtle) changes. If they don't think anything has changed, they may not see the need for additional help. If you, or another family member who isn't with your parent every day, notices changes that require additional help, saying something as simple as, "I noticed Mom couldn't find the bathroom today when I came to visit. When did that start?" may be enough to make the spouse aware of changes — and the need for help.

Some caregivers say the spouse was resistant to any help because it's part of their personality and who they are.

If your parent remains resistant to receiving help — yet is *truly* committed to caring for your parent at home for as long as possible — it may help to ask them to consider that evidence shows placement of a loved one in a nursing home can typically be delayed by up to 1.5 years *simply by the caregiver receiving caregiver services, including counseling, information and ongoing support.*[1]

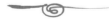

Supporting Mom was our primary concern, especially as Dad's disease progressed. She had very few moments when her mind was free and relaxed. I wish we could

*have gotten her to take time off but she just didn't want to leave Dad. — **Dan***

♡

For two years, my dad did an outstanding job caring for my mom. Slowly, Mom became more demanding and even though Dad tried, she wasn't getting the care she really needed. We also saw Dad's health begin to deteriorate. He lost weight, had terrible diarrhea and was getting little (if any) sleep.

We finally decided to do an intervention. We sat Dad down and told him what we were seeing and demanded he go to his doctor. Prior to the intervention, we had met with his doctor and a nursing home in order to coordinate Dad's admittance to the hospital along with Mom's admittance to a nursing home.

The day we took Mom was very tough. She knew she wouldn't be coming home again and we didn't lie to her when she asked. She cried and Dad did everything he could to delay the process. He kept getting a drink or snack for her or looking for some unnecessary item. None of us wanted to be there but Dad was dehydrated and weak — both physically and emotionally.

We were fortunate that the nursing home was attached to the hospital so we could wheel Mom up to visit my dad. I think that helped ease their separation. By the time Dad was sent home, a few weeks later, it seemed they both realized this was best for both of them. Dad visited Mom daily for about two years but, as she got farther away, you could see his commitment wane and burnout set in. He started hoarding to fill the void and we argued with him over the craziest things. Finally, after about six months, we met with his doctor and told him our concerns. It took a lot of convincing but we were finally able to get Dad to go on antidepressants.

It's been a long road back to some degree of normalcy for him. We are trying to make sure he gets proper nutrition, exercise, and socialization but it is taking a full team

*effort and cooperation. The next step is assisted living —
but we are trying to allow him to be at home as long as
we can. —Jayme*

♡

*Dad has always been strong-willed and likes things to go
his way. So I work around that. I talk to him — constantly. I call every morning to make sure he's okay. Then,
when I get home from work, I call to ask about his day. I
usually call back a few hours later to talk with him and
Mom before they go to bed.*

*When Dad needed to have hip replacement surgery he
was very uneasy about leaving Mom. I talked to my
brother. Together, we told Dad we would take time off
from work so Mom wouldn't be alone. We emphasized the
surgery was important not only so he could continue taking
care of Mom, but so he could play golf (which he loves).*

*During the time Dad was in the hospital and in rehab,
I stayed with Mom. My brother helped on weekends so I
could get a break. When Dad got out of rehab, I stayed at
their house for the first week. After I returned to work, I
went to my parents' house after work to cook them dinner. Friends from our church also helped out but it was
becoming apparent that Dad needed more help. His personality was changing and he wasn't doing some of the
things he'd always enjoyed.*

*When Dad finally admitted he needed help, we started
taking Mom to an adult day center three times a week.
Before long, it became obvious that Dad needed even
more help.*

*We all want to keep Mom home so we now have some-
one from a home-care agency come to my parent's house
twice a week, on the days Mom is home. I do all of my parents' cooking and go up after work and on weekends. My
brother calls or comes up almost every weekend, too.*

*My brother and I encourage Dad to talk to us. We tell
him we understand what he's going through and that we
recognize how difficult it must be but I still sometimes*

wonder how Dad must feel. I see the sadness in his eyes when he looks at Mom or talks about her. He told me recently he doesn't think he could ever take her to a nursing home, leave her there, and walk away. I thank God for that because there is no way I am ready to even think about that. I'll help my dad and do whatever I can so we can keep Mom at home. — **Judy**

My father had been caring for my mom but it was clear that he was burning out. Her needs were outdistancing his abilities and both of them needed daily assistance. My siblings and I knew that his health was in decline and it was compromising his ability to care for Mom long-term.

Although it was difficult, my siblings and I (along with our spouses), approached my father and told him we felt it was time for Mom to get a diagnosis so she could get the best medical care possible. At first, he was reluctant but he found the input of the medical professionals extremely convincing. We all found their advice to be extremely helpful. It also helped my father see the need to move from an independent living scenario to one that was more supportive.

My husband and I moved back to Michigan and, within weeks, Dad and Mom moved into our home and my brother's family — and our family — supported Dad in caring for Mom. — **Shelly**

The Promise

A spouse may also be resistant to outside (or any) help because they made a promise, as many couples do, to always care for one another. The spouse may feel that if they ever stopped caring for your parent — even if only for an afternoon or a day — it would somehow be breaking a sacred promise or dishonoring their marital vows of "in sickness and in health." Sometimes making and attempting to keep such a promise becomes not only unrealistic but unhealthy for the spouse.

Jeannot cared for her husband for over 13 years. She admits her daughter and son "fussed at her" for three years because "they were afraid I was going to die" but Jeannot wanted to honor her promise to her husband — and herself — that she would care for him. When I asked Jeannot how that promise and caring for her husband has impacted her family, she declined to answer. Instead, she suggested I ask her daughters, Rhonda and Sabrina. Following are their individual stories.

My mother has been the primary caregiver and, at times, I have found this to be just as complicated as other aspects of the disease.

Mom promised Dad that she wouldn't put him in a home and, I believe, that promise has cost her. Even when everyone agreed she had more than kept her promise, and that Dad needed care she could no longer provide, she continued to care for him at home. I think Mom had to make sure in her heart that she had given 110% and that's not something her children or anybody should question or interfere with. Instead, I think it's something we should honor.

In the meantime, we did what we could. We listened. We took Mom out as much as we could. We learned what was fun for Mom and what wasn't. Most movies, and certain places or restaurants, were triggers and made her miss Dad, so those were crossed off the list.

We helped around the house, ran errands and did grocery shopping — anything that lessened her burden. My siblings and I talked about what else we could do because we saw that Mom was exhausted.

*For us, a broken ankle finally stopped Mom. Dad went into a home and Mom finally recognized she couldn't care for him any longer. It was her body that finally made the decision for her — otherwise, she would still be caring for Dad. — **Rhonda***

As far as I'm concerned, my mother is a saint. For the past three years, I've seen her go through every emotion there is within a ten-minute timeframe. I tried to prepare her for the possibility of putting Dad in a facility. I talked to whomever would listen and asked for advice on how we could pay for Dad's continued care or how I could convince Mom to let him go. Every time I came up with a solution, Mom would say, "No, I can still do it."

Through the VA, I was able to get Dad into daycare. Instantly, I could see a change in Mom's mood. She was more relaxed. She smiled more. At times, she would say she wished daycare lasted longer but then felt guilty for feeling that way. No matter how hard we tried to tell her we understood, she still felt guilty and wouldn't agree to a permanent move.

My husband and I talked to her about having the two of them move in with us. I was willing to do anything to get Mom some help. I told her, repeatedly, that I had already lost my dad and now I was going to lose my mother, too.

Then Mom fell and broke her ankle in three places. Her injuries required major surgery and an extended stay in the hospital and rehab. Although I felt horrible that she was in so much pain, for the first time I felt I could finally get Mom the help she needed.

I knew she wouldn't be able to care for my father so I found a temporary place for him to allow her time to heal and also let her get used to the idea of having someone else take care of him. When we visited Dad, she was surprised how well he was doing away from home.

I did research on financial aid and while Mom was in rehab, I gave her the information. I knew, ultimately, it would be her decision and I would never have done anything without Mom's consent. I also knew she still needed time to accept the seriousness of her injuries and she needed time to grieve, be alone, get stronger, and still feel in control.

After 20 days, my father was moved into a permanent

facility and, at that point, my mother — while still very much in control — allowed me to start handling the details and making the arrangements for my father's care.

Every now and then when she sees Dad, she'll say, "I still think I could take care of him again." Then she looks at me and says, "Okay, maybe not." — **Sabrina**

Jeannot admits she "was on overload to the point that I didn't even see it myself" and that "breaking my ankle finally forced all the issues to the forefront. I'm still sleeping many hours to regain 'me'."

How Can A Son or Daughter Help?

Many caregivers share the same concerns as Rhonda and Sabrina. Over time, they become increasingly concerned about the health and welfare of both their parents. Many also struggle with knowing how to adequately support their parent who was the primary caregiver.

I asked one of our caregivers, Kitty, about this. Kitty has cared for both a parent and a husband with Alzheimer's. This affords her the ability to view caregiving from the perspective of both a daughter and a spouse. I asked Kitty to place herself in the role of the spouse and to imagine she received a letter from her daughters asking what they could do to support her as the caregiver. Here is Kitty's reply:

Dear Girls:

I received your note today. First, I want to tell you how much I appreciate everything you've done for your father and me over these past few difficult years. You're right when you say that things are getting a little more "difficult" but, at the same time, things are just "different" and, in some ways, are getting a little easier. Let me try to explain.

The near-constant physical attention and supervision Dad now requires with dressing, feeding, etc. can be exhausting for both of us. As his ability to communicate also continues to decline, I find myself becoming very frustrated in trying to understand what he wants or needs. He can be so childish at times and it reminds me of when you were young. The sad difference is that I knew you would grow out of your dependence on me while Dad only grows more dependent.

On the brighter side (if there is such a thing), Dad is now at the point with the disease where he isn't as argumentative as he was early on. His mood swings aren't as dramatic, his medications seem more effective, he finally sleeps better and he smiles more. Perhaps the blessing in all of this (again, if there is one) is that he has now reached the stage in this painful progression where he is no longer consciously aware of his own loss of self. How terribly frightening it must be to lose one's self. I take some degree of sad comfort in no longer seeing the fear in his eyes that I once saw.

You ask what you can do for me.

Please don't criticize me if I tell you the time has come when I can no longer meet all of his physical and emotional needs alone. I have been exploring all the options available to me for quite some time now and I can assure you that whatever decision I make will be a thoughtful and deliberate one.

Please respect my decisions. While I greatly value your thoughts and opinions, understand I have a very different perspective than you. I've tried over the years to be as open and honest as I can about your father's condition. However, from time to time, I've had to make decisions I know you didn't fully understand or appreciate (for example, when I took his car away and cancelled his credit cards). As tough as these decisions were, they were made for his (and my) protection. Know it's hard enough to make these difficult decisions without having to defend them, too.

Please know I take my responsibility to your father very seriously. However, your father and I learned one important thing as we watched your grandfather devote himself wholly to your grandmother's care. During your grandmother's progression into what I now call the "abyss of Alzheimer's," your grandfather became a tragic prisoner of care. Both your father and I shared the belief that, at some point, that kind of so-called "unselfish devotion" only becomes martyrdom. Your father didn't want that for either of us.

No one can say how long this hiatus from "real life" will be, but I know, from experience, it is temporary. I do have a life I am anxious to get back to but, in the meantime, promise me, you will speak up and tell me if you think I'm becoming the martyr.

Please come and visit as often as you want — and stay as long as you can. I know at times, when you visit Dad, it may seem like you're talking to a stranger or that he doesn't know you at all. Trust me, he does know you — and loves you very much.

And know that I always look forward to your visits — and that I love you, too.

Hugs,
Mom

Keep In Touch With the Outside World

You may find, as the disease progresses and your parent's behavior changes, that friends and family stop visiting. This is no one's fault. Much of this is human nature and a natural response to the disease. People often fear or shy away from things they don't understand and Alzheimer's is difficult for many people to understand.

However, human contact and interaction with others is important for your parent and you. You can keep in touch through phone calls, e-mail, letters or cards but, chances are, your parent can't. Therefore, consider inviting and encouraging friends and family to visit even if your parent no longer remembers them. Remind the person that while Alzheimer's may have changed your parent's memory, it hasn't changed the fact that they, and their friendship, are still important to your family.

If a person wants to visit but seems hesitant, it may be

because they aren't sure what to say or how to act around your parent. Assure them you will help them or you can prepare them in advance of the visit. Tell them to:

- ❑ Call your parent by their first name.
- ❑ Not take it personally if your parent doesn't recognize them or call them by name. Explain they may have to remind your parent more than once what their name is — and to do so without making a big deal out of it.
- ❑ Remain calm and talk quietly if your parent gets confused, angry or upset.
- ❑ Avoid physical contact (hugs, handshakes or getting too close) until they know how your parent will react.
- ❑ Consider bringing along a photo album, music or an activity to do with your parent.
- ❑ Tell the person that if, on the day of their visit, your parent is having a difficult day you will advise them and discuss the possibility of rescheduling their visit.

Arrange visits at the time of day that is best for your parent. If mornings are when your mother is least agitated, invite someone over for morning coffee. Make sure you limit the number of people who visit at one time as the noise or confusion may be upsetting for your parent.

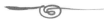

PART THREE: Caring for Yourself

> *"Over fifty million caregivers spend every spare minute driving to medical appointments, stopping at the pharmacy, cooking, answering questions, paying bills, and helping with matters that used to be private. They feel trapped in an endless loop and need to release the stress of caregiving."* — **B. Lynn Goodwin, author of *"You Want Me To Do What?: Journaling for Caregivers"***

Caregivers are sometimes called the hidden or silent victims of Alzheimer's. With the focus typically being on the individual with

Alzheimer's, oftentimes others — and the caregivers themselves — forget the disease is impacting them as well. In order for you to continue providing care for your parent over the long haul it's critical that, *first and foremost*, you take care of yourself. Caring for yourself isn't optional and is perhaps one of the most important parts of your journey.

Your life is probably a juggling act. In addition to caring for your parent, you may be supporting your other parent as the primary caregiver — or *you* may be the primary caregiver. And then there are all the other pieces of your life.

Cooking, cleaning, mortgage payments and kids' soccer games don't magically disappear just because you are caring for your parent. Children go off to college, marital and financial difficulties arise, and illness or death can — and quite often does — occur. Real life doesn't stop for Alzheimer's.

Caring for a parent with Alzheimer's has some very unique challenges — and stressors. More than 40 percent of family and other unpaid caregivers rate the emotional stress of caring for an individual with Alzheimer's as high or very high.[2]

Take care of yourself. Don't become a silent victim of Alzheimer's.

Ask For — and Accept — Help

One of the most important — and sometimes most difficult — parts of caring for your parent is asking for help. However, it's important that you remain realistic. Caring for a parent with Alzheimer's is a long, exhausting journey and no one can, or should be expected to, do it alone or without help.

It's important to be willing to ask for — and accept — help. It's equally important, when asking for help, to ask for *specific* help. Rather than saying "I need help" say, "I would like to take a yoga class on Tuesday afternoons. Can you stay with Mom?" or "The next time you go to the grocery store, could you pick up a gallon of milk for us?" Sometimes people don't help because they don't know exactly what it is you need or what they can do. By being specific, it takes away any guesswork for the other person since they know exactly how they can help. Being specific also increases your chance of getting the help — and break — you need.

For more guidance with this, see *Appendix B: Finding Support, Getting Help: An Exercise* in the *Resource* section of this book.

Take Time for Yourself

With so many things demanding your immediate attention, it may seem impossible to find time for yourself. Caregivers say to begin with a small, manageable amount of time: one minute.

Taking a one minute break doesn't require you to physically leave your parent's side. While your dad is eating his breakfast or your mom is getting dressed, allow yourself to *mentally* step aside to:

- **Breathe.** All of us have a tendency when we are stressed to breathe faster (or not at all). The simple act of taking a few deep, slow breaths can decrease anxiety and tension and help with mental clarity.
- **Count Backwards.** Starting at 20, slowly (and silently) count backwards to zero. This helps take the focus off whatever may have been crowding or clouding your mind and, instead, forces you into a calmer state.
- **Count Your Blessings.** For one minute think of nothing other than the blessings in your life and the things for which you are grateful.

Many caregivers say that, after paying attention to their day, they were able to find longer periods of time, perhaps while their parent was engrossed in a TV show or taking a nap, to:

- Read, write or journal.
- Take a walk around the yard or sit outside.
- Sit quietly with a cup of tea.
- Listen to music.
- Watch a sunset.
- Knit or crochet.
- Meditate or pray.
- Take a bubble bath.

While getting away for an afternoon, an entire day, or longer will require more advanced planning, caregivers say it's worth the effort. Giving yourself a period of time to step out of your role as caregiver allows you to regroup and refocus. It will also give you time to replenish and refresh your body, mind and spirit so you can return to your parent a calmer, more relaxed caregiver. Caregiving can also take a toll on the other relationships in your life so scheduling time away with your spouse, a child, or close friend can also help you renew those connections.

Sometimes, taking time means nothing more than unplugging the phone or learning to pace yourself. With so much to do each day, it may be tempting to think the more or faster you go, the better off you'll be. Slow down…pace yourself…and breathe.

Take Care of Your Health

Studies show that family and unpaid caregivers of individuals with Alzheimer's are more likely than unpaid caregivers of individuals without Alzheimer's to say that caregiving made their health worse[3,4]

Many caregivers say it wasn't until after their parent died that they realized just how much they had ignored their own health — and that it took years to regain even a portion of their health back.

It's critical to take care of your own health not only for yourself but for your parent. If you get sick, the entire caregiving "machine" may come to a grinding halt and, rather than taking time to recuperate, you may be trying to find (and manage) others who can step in to take care of your parent.

You can help ensure your ongoing health by:

❑ Getting a regular check-up.

❑ Eating a healthy, balanced diet. Don't skip meals.

❑ Taking a good multi-vitamin every day.

❑ Watching your intake of sugar, coffee or caffeinated beverages or an excess of carbohydrates. They can leave you feeling run down, tired, jittery or irritable.

❑ Exercising. This doesn't mean you have to go to a gym. Exercise can be something you enjoy and that fits into your day — perhaps going for a walk with your parent, gardening, or turning on some music and dancing!

❑ Learning to relax
❑ Getting enough sleep.

RELAXATION AND SLEEP TIPS

Learning to relax and get enough sleep are critical to your ongoing physical and mental well-being. For many caregivers, operating in high-alert or crisis mode all day, every day, becomes quite normal. However, you can't operate in "crisis mode" constantly — or for very long. Your body will eventually catch up with you and you'll find yourself feeling even more overwhelmed, exhausted and depleted. And, even though your body may be exhausted, you may find it difficult to unwind and get a good night's sleep. It may be helpful to create a bedtime ritual that encourages and enhances a good night's sleep.

• Take a warm bath or shower. Use lavender-scented soap or body wash.

• Sip a cup of relaxing tea (perhaps with chamomile or lemon balm).

• Write in a journal to release any leftover or pent-up emotions or frustrations from the day. If possible, try to end your writing session by switching to writing about the blessings — rather than the difficulties — of the day.

• Meditate or pray to quiet your mind, release negative thinking, reduce anxiety and turn your concerns over to a "higher power."

• Make sure your space is conducive to sleep. Turn off televisions, cell phones and computers. Turn clocks with digital displays so the display isn't facing your bed (or cover it with a scarf). The artificial light from these objects can be misread by your brain as daylight, thereby not allowing your body to relax and prepare for sleep.

• As much as possible, try to stick to a regular bedtime.

• If all else fails, try taking catnaps during the day. Some sleep is better than no sleep.

Express Your Feelings

Caring for a parent with Alzheimer's can bring a cacophony of emotions: confusion, sadness, anger, frustration, exhaustion. All of these feelings are normal but they can also build up and result in a caregiver becoming overwhelmed or burned out.

It's important to express your feelings. Find a friend, relative, another caregiver, or a support group who you can safely and comfortably share your feelings with. Some caregivers also sought the services of a professional therapist or counselor.

For many caregivers, keeping a journal allowed them to vent feelings and emotions that might otherwise have remained bottled up. A journal can also be a tool for you to find new levels of acceptance, and comfort, both now and in the future.

By keeping a journal, you may begin to see the healing power of words. Expressing what you're feeling in your journal can help diminish the stress of a situation and allow you to maintain a positive outlook. Journaling can be a way to heal your mind and soul as you struggle through the difficult days with Alzheimer's.

When Dad was first diagnosed, I thought as long as I kept Dad's life as normal as possible, we could beat the disease. I wrote in my journal every day about what he was doing. As I went back and read what I'd already written, I began to see that Dad was digressing which allowed me to accept that I was never going to cure him.

Now, when I read the words I wrote back then, I remember things so clearly. I remember the confusion and ugliness of the situation but I also see how I held onto hope. I see how writing in my journal enabled me to keep things in perspective. I see how I constantly asked God for help in caring for Dad. It wasn't until after Dad died, and I read my journal again, that I saw how God had held and helped me every step of the way.

Marie Fostino is a former caregiver and the author of "Alzheimer's: A Caretaker's Journal."

Be Gentle With Yourself

We can sometimes be our own worst critics. We often set the bar extraordinarily high for ourselves and are completely unrealistic in our expectations of ourselves. We sometimes look back and see how we could have done things differently — and with better results. As a result, we may blame ourselves, or feel guilty, for what we could — or should — have done for our parent.

Blaming yourself or feeling guilty can be destructive to your psyche. Remember that loving and caring for your parent is a journey — and, generally, a very long journey. It's only natural that you will learn things along the way: new ways to handle a situation or behavior or new ways to care for your parent or yourself. That doesn't mean you failed yourself — or your parent — in the past. It means you did the very best you could based on the information you had at the time. It also means you are learning and growing as a caregiver — and a person — and that's a good, a very good, thing.

So please don't judge yourself. Instead, honor all that you are doing as you love and care for yourself. Be proud of all you've accomplished thus far. Be good to yourself. Be gentle with yourself.

SIGNS OF CAREGIVER BURN-OUT

Put a check next to any of the following that may apply to you.

On a regular basis, do you, or any other caregiver:

❑ Have difficulty sleeping?

❑ Find yourself withdrawn from family and friends?

❑ Have trouble focusing or concentrating?

❑ Cry frequently and often without reason?

❑ Deny to others that there's anything wrong?

❑ No longer participate in activities that you once enjoyed?

❑ Feel sad, depressed, or hopeless?

❑ Feel overwhelmed or that you have the weight of the world on your shoulders?

❑ Find yourself easily frustrated, angry or irritable with your parent or others?

❑ Find yourself having increased problems with your physical health?

- ❏ Feel anxious about today (or the future)?
- ❏ Feel exhausted or having difficult completing simple, daily tasks?
- ❏ Find your mind won't stop spinning? Can't stop thinking?
- ❏ Be honest about your intake of alcohol and prescription or over-the-counter medicine.
- ❏ Are you consuming more and more coffee in an attempt to get (or maintain) your energy?

If you answered "Yes" to any of these, it may indicate you are experiencing symptoms of "caregiver burnout" and may be putting your own health at risk. Take a break. If the symptoms continue, consider talking with your doctor or professional.

Studies indicate that when a caregiver receives help and support they are better able to care for their parent — and the longer their parent is able to remain at home.

Chapter 5

A Journey of "What-Ifs"

Since Alzheimer's isn't logical or predictable, one of the biggest difficulties Alzheimer's caregivers face is knowing how or what to prepare for. This was probably best expressed by a dear friend of mine one day when we met for lunch.

"I read about the different phases and all the signs indicated that the next thing we should prepare for was wandering," she said. "So I got myself and the house ready but, instead, Dad started hallucinating. And I wasn't ready for that. Honestly, I don't know what to prepare for. I might get ready for one thing but what if it turns out to be something else I should have prepared for. I just don't know if I'm ready for this. It's all the "what- ifs" that scare me the most."

In this chapter, caregivers will give you ideas and tips — as well as courage and confidence — to help you face all the "what-ifs." We'll begin with the "what-if" most caregivers say you should take care of first: ensuring your parent's safety.

PART ONE: All The "What-Ifs"
Think Safety First

The first thing I would address would be matters of safety.
— Jeannot

Safety should be every caregiver's primary concern because, as time passes, your parent's filters and ability to discern what is appropriate or safe will disappear. Therefore, it is up to you to take the necessary steps to ensure their current, and continued, well-being and safety.

Safety At Home

We'll begin by looking at your parent's home environment. Whether your parent is living independently, with a family member, or in a facility, it's important to look at their home environment through *their* eyes. Consider what might be dangerous, confusing or stressful from *their* perspective.

In many ways, it's similar to child-proofing a home. However, unlike a child who can be taught about safety, your parent can't and won't. Therefore, it's up to you to remove, change or replace any unsafe items and put systems in place to ensure their current and continued safety.

❑ Acknowledge and accept the fact that your parent cannot be left alone. If your parent is living alone, or is left alone for extended periods of time, have someone check on them regularly throughout the day.

❑ Place important phone numbers — emergency numbers, medical personnel and family members — next to every phone. There are telephones you can buy that will make using a telephone easier for your parent.

❑ Have a system in place so that, should your parent fall or need help, they can send for, and receive, help without the use of a telephone.

❑ Devise a system of safely storing and dispensing your parent's medication.

❑ Remove, lock up, or put out of reach, any and all chemicals or toxic products including household cleaning products, alcohol, guns, hunting equipment, knives, scissors or other sharp instruments.

❑ Put any outdoor items that could be a potential danger — such as saws, lighter fluid, power tools, pesticides and paint — in a locked garage or tool shed.

❑ Remove, lock up or put out of reach any potential fire or burn hazards (candles, lighters, matches, toaster, toaster oven, iron, curling irons, small heaters, etc.).

❑ Set the temperature on the hot water heater and install anti-scald devices on faucets and shower heads.

❑ Disconnect the stove or install safety knobs or an automatic shut-off switch on the stove to prevent burns or fires.

❑ Install child-safety covers on electrical outlets and child-safety latches on all kitchen cabinets and drawers.

❑ Install alarms on all outside windows and doors.

❑ Install handrails on all stairways (both inside and outside the home).

❑ Install grab bars in the bathtub and next to the toilet.

❑ Keep the home well-lit, especially at night. Waking up in total darkness can disorient an Alzheimer's patient.

❑ Consider removing locks on bathroom and bedroom doors to avoid the possibility your parent could accidentally lock themselves in and not be able to get out.

❑ Remove area rugs or clutter that could cause a fall.

❑ Remove any loose items on tables, such as table runners and placemats.

❑ Remove poisonous plants and any small objects that could cause choking.

❑ Decorate with solid colors, whenever possible, since patterns can sometimes be confusing for someone with Alzheimer's.

❑ Make sure there is adequate lighting, both inside and out-side the home. Use nightlights since waking up in total darkness can be disorienting or upsetting to your parent.

❑ If your parent lives independently and smokes, try remov-ing ash trays, matches, or anything smoking-related that could remind them to smoke. If your parent lives with you, consider placing a non-flammable apron over them when they are smoking to prevent burns. Know there will come a time when your parent will no longer be able to smoke unattended.

❑ Have smoke alarms, carbon monoxide detectors and fire extinguishers in the home. Make sure they are easily acces-sible and check them regularly to ensure they are working properly.

A NOTE ON CHILD-SAFETY DEVICES, LOCKS AND LATCHES

Consider the following when using child-safety devices or installing locks on windows and doors:

• Don't assume that child-safety devices are foolproof. While your parent's behavior may be childlike, they still have the strength of an adult and may also have the ingenuity to fig-ure out a child-safety device, thereby making it ineffective.

• All locks and latches on doors and windows should be installed at a height where your parent can't reach or access them. Some caregivers say their parent only sees (or fiddles with) things at eye level so installing locks high up, or down low, helped.

• Keep in mind that locks on doors and windows can prohibit you — *and emergency personnel* — from entering the house. Make sure whatever locks you install permit some-one to access the house within minutes in the event of an emergency.

• If installing locks that require the use of a key, make sure someone outside the home has copies of the keys (and consider leaving a set with your local police).

Safety During a Mandatory Evacuation

Another caregiver shared insights into something many of us might never consider: keeping your parent safe during a government-declared mandatory evacuation.

One of the "what-ifs" I found challenging was what to do in case of a government-declared mandatory evacuation.

Following Hurricanes Katrina and Rita, the assisted living facility where my husband resided required every family to execute a document stating the family would be responsible for getting the patient out of the facility — and also released the facility from any responsibility for my husband's care — during such an emergency. Until then, I had no idea that nursing homes/assisted living facilities often will not accept responsibility for a patient's care or transportation during a government-declared mandatory evacuation.

I was fortunate to find a sister-facility 400 miles inland that agreed to take my husband in the event of such an evacuation but I still had the problem of how to get my husband there. I entered into a contract with the assisted living facility where my husband lived in which they agreed to provide a private-duty nurse/companion who would accompany my husband. I was responsible for making arrangements for all flight and ground transportation for both my husband and the nurse. In addition I was to pay round-trip air transportation for both of them as well as the standard hourly rate for the nurse. The sister facility agreed to pick up my husband and the nurse at the airport and guaranteed my husband availability at one of their facilities at the per diem rate I was paying at his current facility.

Gratefully, I only had to partially implement the plan once but I learned, in order for it to be successful, it had to be implemented within 72 hours of an impending emergency. During Hurricane Ike, my husband's home facility was damaged and without electricity for 16 days but he had died three months earlier. — *Kitty*

Communication

As Alzheimer's progresses, it may become increasingly difficult for your parent to express their thoughts or communicate. They may also have difficulty understanding what you, or others, are trying to tell them. While there are no guaranteed methods to ensure everything you say will be understood by your parent, or vice versa, caregivers say the following helped enhance communication between them and their parent.

- ❏ Use short, simple sentences and words.
- ❏ Try to ask questions that can be answered with a simple "yes" or "no."
- ❏ Only ask one question at a time.
- ❏ Use visuals or demonstrate, when possible, to help your parent understand what you are saying. For example, if you're asking them if they'd like an apple or a pear, show them both fruits to help them understand and decide.
- ❏ It's not just what you say but how you say it. Stay calm, be positive, be patient.
- ❏ Speak slowly and quietly. Avoid raising your voice.
- ❏ Be aware of your body language and the tone of your voice.
- ❏ If your parent is struggling to find a word and you know what they're trying to say, help them.
- ❏ Be patient and allow your parent sufficient time to process what you are saying.
- ❏ Remain at eye level with them.
- ❏ Make eye contact and make sure you have your parent's attention. Make sure they are listening before you talk.
- ❏ Understand that sometimes your parent's words may not indicate what they really mean. Watch their body language or non-verbal cues for the real meaning behind their words.
- ❏ If your parent doesn't understand, try repeating or re-phrasing the sentence or question. If it's not important, and you can do so without upsetting them, try changing the subject.

❏ Stop and listen. Show them you're interested in — and are trying to understand — what they are saying.

❏ Don't interrupt your parent and avoid arguing or criticizing them.

❏ Don't boss your parent around. Instead, give them options or choices in a positive manner and voice.

❏ If you're unable to convey a message with words alone, you can sometimes get your parent to understand through touch. When I had trouble getting Mom to lift her leg to put her pants on, I would touch her foot as I asked her to lift her leg. It worked like a charm.

❏ Call your parent by name and, if necessary, remind them of your name and who you are.

❏ If you simply can't understand what they are saying, a simple apology can work wonders.

One additional suggestion (and something I learned from my father) is to avoid having upsetting conversations in front of your parent. I remember a few instances where people offered my father suggestions on how to care for my mother — while Mom was sitting at the table with them. My father was adamant about not having conversations in front of my mother that could upset her so he would get up and walk away or out of the room. When he returned, he would simply say, "Don't act like she's not in the room or doesn't exist. She's right here and understands — probably more than we can imagine."

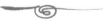

When she used the wrong word, Mom would make a joke of it and laugh. We followed her cue and laughed, too. We tried to be very careful to never laugh at Mom or say anything that would hurt her feelings.

My husband, Carl, learned about being careful what you say one evening when I was out with some friends and Carl was home with Mom.

As it was getting late, Carl told Mom it was time to go to bed. Mom just sat there looking at him.

"Come on, Mom," Carl said. "Let's go to bed."

Mom got up and followed him into the kitchen but as they neared the bedrooms, she stopped, turned to him and said, "Carl, I think the world of you but..."

Luckily, Carl caught on and pointed Mom towards her bedroom, assuring her he was going the opposite way to our bedroom. He now understand that things have changed and he has to be very careful of how and what he says to Mom. — *Bonnie*

My grandmother communicated fairly well until the very end. After she had several strokes, speech became a problem and certain words were difficult for her. I remember one time she couldn't say "computer." She kept stuttering and struggling, and finally slammed her fists down and just gave up. I think she may have been embarrassed to ask for help at times so we asked her regularly if she was thirsty, hungry, or needed to use the bathroom. — *Cassie*

After a while there wasn't a lot of verbal communication. Mom would try so hard to search for words and then would just stop talking. But there are other ways to communicate. A hug would make her feel better if she was frustrated or agitated. — *Dorothy*

Listen and ask questions in a loving manner. Assure your parent that all is well. My dad can't distinguish dreams from reality. He worries he's going to jail, is missing an appointment, or that no one loves him. I reassure him, hug him and hold his hand to calm him down. — *Wanda*

PERSONAL HYGIENE: Dressing, Bathing and Toileting

For the majority of people, matters of personal hygiene are private activities. For those with Alzheimer's, due to the disorientation and confusion that accompany the disease, others often have to assist them, thereby making personal hygiene tasks difficult and sometimes impossible for you and your parent. We'll begin with what our caregivers felt was the least invasive and problematic: Dressing.

Dressing

Caregivers say many problems with dressing can be avoided by following these tips:

- ❑ Limit your parent's choices. Don't open the closet door and ask your parent what they'd like to wear. If possible, choose their outfit for them.

- ❑ If your parent insists on choosing their outfit, lay out one or two coordinating outfits (making sure all tops and bottoms match).

- ❑ Hand your parent one article of clothing at a time and in the order in which they should be put on.

- ❑ Loose fitting and easy-on/easy-off clothing is best. Choose clothing with minimal (or no) belts, buckles, buttons and zippers. Clothing with Velcro and elastic waists — as well as slip-on shoes and tube socks — are best.

- ❑ Be available to provide guidance and instructions, if needed, but allow and encourage your parent to dress themselves for as long as possible.

- ❑ Don't rush your parent. Like everything else, getting dressed will take much longer than it normally would. Be patient.

- ❑ Don't argue with your parent if his or her clothes don't match or they want to wear the same thing over and over again. As long as their clothes are clean, it really doesn't matter. Your day will go much smoother if you choose your battles wisely.

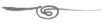

- After my grandmother started having mini-strokes, she lost the ability to use her arms and legs and we had to help her get dressed. My mother and grandfather found it easiest to dress her in button-up shirts and stretch pants. — *Cassie*

- Mom often layered her clothes. Sometimes she wore two or three shirts and a couple pairs of pants. Unless I thought she would be too hot, it was never a problem because it was important for her to feel independent for as long as she could. — *Dorothy*

Bathing

Bathing and problems surrounding bathing can be caused (or escalated) by a combination of things that might be affecting your parent including physical illness, inadequate lighting, lack of privacy, the room or water being too hot or cold, fear of water or falling, or no longer understanding the reason behind (or necessity for) a bath or getting their hair washed.

The following steps, suggested by our caregivers, helped alleviate some problems surrounding bathing.

- ❑ Make sure the tub area is safe. Place non-slip mats or adhesive decals inside (and outside) the tub.
- ❑ Install grab bars to allow safe, easy access in and out of the tub. Don't rely on towel racks for stability or safety.
- ❑ If mobility is an issue for your parent, consider using a bath chair. Since the chair also sits above the water, it may also make your parent feel comfortable and safe.
- ❑ Be prepared. Get the room and bath ready in advance. Make sure you have everything you need ready and available — towels, bathrobe, shampoo and soap.
- ❑ Make sure the temperature of the room and water is comfortable and that there is adequate lighting.
- ❑ Allow your parent to feel the water in advance of getting in. This may help reassure and relax them.
- ❑ Avoid lengthy explanations or discussions about the bath. Break the bathing process into small, easily-understood tasks. (Rather than saying "Mom, it's time to take a bath and wash your hair" say "Okay, Mom, let's take your shoes and socks off" or "Feel the water, Dad.")
- ❑ Avoid arguing over the necessity to bathe. Arguing can add to your parent's agitation. Instead, keep them focused on the individual task at hand. Your parent may switch their focus and forget they were arguing with you.
- ❑ Stay consistent with your parent's typical bathing routine. If they always took baths don't try to have them take

showers. Sometimes the change in routine may be what's upsetting them.

❑ Use your parent's favorite shampoo or scent.

❑ Avoid using perfumed soaps, bath oil or bubble bath since Alzheimer's patients can be quite susceptible to urinary tract infections. Also avoid using talcum powder in the groin area. Instead try a talc-free, unscented powder or cornstarch. Cornstarch is inexpensive, non-allergenic and odorless.

❑ If your parent remains agitated, upset, nervous or angry, try giving them a bath at another time.

❑ Sometimes having water poured over their head may upset your parent. If you always wash their hair when they take a bath, they may equate a bath with getting their hair washed and get agitated. Try doing the two things separately.

❑ Choose a time of day when your parent is the most relaxed and least agitated.

❑ If modesty or privacy might be the concern for your parent, make sure curtains, blinds and doors are closed. In the tub, try putting a towel around them to further respect their need for privacy. Likewise, hold a towel in front of them when they are getting in and out of the bathtub or have towel and bathrobe ready so they can cover up.

❑ Give your parent a washcloth or something to hold.

❑ Play soft music.

❑ Consider using aromatherapy. Spraying the towels or room with lavender may help relax them.

❑ Don't leave your parent alone! Not for a second!

❑ If bathing continues to be an ongoing problem, consider other forms of bathing. Caregivers say it's not critical your parent get a full bath every day. Supplement with sponge, no-rinse or towel baths. (For more information on towel baths and other creative bathing techniques, see *Bathing Without A Battle* in the *Resource* section).

- Mom often didn't realize she hadn't bathed in a couple of days so gentle reminders were best — and generally worked. — *Ann*

- Mom went from a cleaning fanatic and someone who ironed her underwear to not wanting to take a bath — ever. There was a period where she was actually scared to even be in the shower. One day, I got into the shower fully-clothed just to show her it was safe. Mom laughed so hard but, after that, her anxiety dissipated. — *Dorothy*

- Dad was able to wash his face and brush his teeth but, since he often left the water running in the sink, we installed a control that automatically shut the water off. We also had some success with sponge baths, pre-moistened washcloths and shampoo-in-a-cap. — *Frank*

- I had a bath chair in the tub and would get the water ready. Then I would tell Dad I had taken my bath and now it was his turn. I kept the door slightly ajar so I could see if he actually got in the tub or just splashed water on his face. — *Marie*

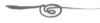

Toileting

Toileting issues and, in particular, incontinence (either urinary or bowel) can be upsetting to your parent — and you. There are a number of possible underlying causes or factors behind incontinence, including: health problems (infection, prostate problem, constipation, weak pelvic muscles, side effect of medication, or a chronic illness such as diabetes, Parkinson's or a stroke) or environmental factors (poor lighting, your parent is restrained or otherwise unable to get out of bed, or the bathroom is just too far away and your parent is unable to get there in time). It could also be your parent no longer recognizes or knows where the bathroom is located, is having difficulty undressing or wiping, is fearful (or embarrassed) to undress in front of a caregiver or staff member, or doesn't know how to tell you they have to go.

Caregivers say taking some simple precautionary steps helped ensure that accidents either didn't happen or, at the very least, limited the possibility. These included:

- ❑ Don't wait for your parent to tell you they have to go to the bathroom. By then, it's usually too late. Watch for indicators such as fidgeting, tugging at their clothes or general restlessness.

- ❑ Establish a routine and take your parent to the bathroom — or remind them — on a regular basis. Caregivers suggest every two to three hours. Also have them sit on the toilet before and after meals and before bed.

- ❑ Install grab bars next to the toilet to help your parent sit down and get up.

- ❑ Consider installing a raised toilet seat with grab bars that lock securely into place.

- ❑ Paint or put a sign or picture on the bathroom door to make it easily recognizable by your parent. The problem may be they simply no longer recognize where the bathroom is located.

- ❑ Make sure there is adequate lighting for your parent to find the bathroom.

- ❑ Consider placing a commode next to (or near) their bed for use during the night.

- ❑ Be mindful and listen for other words your parent may use, like *leak, pee* or *tinkle* and make sure all caregivers are aware of all words that signal they need to use the bathroom.

- ❑ Clothes that are easy for your parent to put on and take off will make the entire process much easier for them.

- ❑ Limit liquids after 6 PM (or earlier depending upon what time your parent goes to bed). Especially avoid drinks that could have a diuretic effect such as tea, coffee or beer.

- ❑ Many caregivers suggest putting waterproof covers or protective pads on beds and chairs. A few, however, said that having pads on beds or chairs tended to signal to their parent to go to the bathroom. Find what works for you and your parent.

❑ Before going out make sure your parent goes (or at least tries to go) to the bathroom.

❑ When going to an unfamiliar or new place (store, home, restaurant), locate the restrooms as soon as you arrive. If you switch to adult disposable-type undergarments, continue doing all of the above but also make sure to check the undergarment frequently. Staying in wet or soiled undergarments is not only uncomfortable for your parent but can also lead to more serious health conditions.

❑ Keep a travel bag in your car with wipes, a complete change of clothes (including undergarments), disposable undergarments and a plastic bag for any wet/soiled clothing.

❑ Incontinence issues typically don't arise until the latter stages of the disease. If your parent is exhibiting signs of incontinence early on, talk with your doctor to rule out the possibility of an infection or other underlying physical cause.

❑ Keep a toilet snake handy. One caregiver said her parent tried to flush diapers and "virtually everything and anything" down the toilet. Purchasing a snake saved their family on recurrent plumbing bills.

IF YOUR PARENT HAS A TOILETING ACCIDENT

• Stay calm, reassuring, loving and supportive.

• Change your parent's clothes immediately. Don't let your parent get used to the feeling of being in wet or soiled clothes — or think it is normal.

• Wash your parent's skin immediately to avoid rashes or sores.

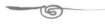

We finally had to go to adult disposable diapers — not the most wonderful thing. The problem after we switched was that I'd find wet diapers in with her clean clothes. She didn't seem to understand they were disposable. — *Ann*

In the later stages of her disease, my grandmother began to wet herself since she couldn't make it to the bathroom very fast. We took two approaches to the situation. First, we would have her sit on the commode several times throughout the day to prevent any accidents. Next, we began to use adult disposable diapers, especially when going out into public. — *Cassie*

When Mom was still able to walk, we took her to the bathroom frequently. — *Dorothy*

Toileting became an issue because Mom didn't remember she had just gone and was going into the bathroom every ten minutes. — *Gayle*

Providing Adequate Nutrition

While providing proper and adequate nutrition is essential to your parent's physical and mental well-being, doing so can be a struggle.

Some caregivers say their parent wanted to eat constantly, either because they had a voracious appetite or because they'd forgotten they already ate. The far greater majority of caregivers were at the opposite end of the spectrum. For them, ensuring their parent received adequate nutrition and hydration was an ongoing battle.

Some individuals with Alzheimer's forget to eat or drink so, for them, a simple reminder or making food available may eliminate the problem. For others, medication either decreases their appetite or makes food taste "funny." All of this is further complicated as the disease progresses, since your parent may no longer remember how, or have the ability, to chew or swallow.

Poor nutrition can result in weight loss, physical weakness, sleeplessness, disorientation, increased irritability, or physical ailments which only add to the litany of problems your parent (and you) may already be juggling.

Caregivers suggest the following:

❏ Keep mealtimes calm and quiet. Avoid noise, distractions or interruptions at mealtime. Turn off the radio, television, and telephones (including cell phones).

❏ If possible, keep a routine and regular time for meals.

❏ Try providing smaller meals throughout the day rather than the typical three large meals.

❏ Provide healthy snacks throughout the day (such as small pieces of fruit, cheese or protein bars) in a consistent location.

❏ Limit the number of foods you put on your parent's plate to avoid confusing or overwhelming them.

❏ Allow extra time for meals.

❏ Remove distractions from the table such as centerpieces or flowers.

❏ Avoid patterned placemats or tablecloths, which can be confusing or distracting for an Alzheimer's patient.

❏ Brightly colored plates may help your parent distinguish between the food and the plate. However, avoid using plates or dishes with patterns as this may be confusing or distracting for your parent.

❏ Sit down and eat with your parent. Try to make mealtime an enjoyable, relaxing time.

❏ Don't be concerned about table manners. The focus isn't on neatness but on allowing your parent to eat independently as long as possible and to keep them well-nourished.

❏ As the disease progresses, your parent may lose all table manners. They may eat from other people's plates, eat with their hands, or eat anything in sight (including items not intended to be eaten). When your parent reaches this stage, you (or another family member) may want to sit and help your parent during mealtime.

❏ When utensils become difficult for your parent to use, cut their food or switch to finger foods. If they are having difficulty holding a glass, try using a straw or switch to a child's sippy-type cup.

❑ If chewing or swallowing becomes a problem, cut your parent's food into small bite-size pieces or switch to soft foods and high-protein shakes.

❑ Nutritious high-calorie snacks and shakes can help if weight loss continues to be a problem.

❑ If weight gain is a concern, keep low-calorie nutritious snacks and fresh fruits and vegetables available.

❑ Keep your parent hydrated.

❑ If your parent has dentures, you may want to have the fit checked. Ill-fitting dentures could make eating painful for your parent.

❑ Check with your parent's doctor to make sure your parent's appetite isn't being caused by their medication or another health condition (such as depression, digestive problems, diabetes or heart disease).

If your other parent is the primary caregiver, you may have concerns whether they have the time, energy or skills to prepare a proper meal and adequate nutrition. You may want to look for additional ways to provide healthy meals for both of your parents. Friends, neighbors, and church members may be willing (and happy) to provide meals that can either be eaten that day or frozen. You can also contact your local Meals on Wheels (or a similar program) which can provide regular, wholesome meals to one (or both) of your parents.

When Mom moved into a local nursing home, I gave the staff all kinds of instructions, including all of her likes and dislikes. I told them she wouldn't drink water or tea and always wanted soda with her meals. I also told them she never ate cheese or anything that contained cheese. A week later, I visited Mom at lunchtime and there she sat enjoying a glass of tea and eating a pimento cheese sandwich — and loving it! I guess she forgot she didn't like those things. — *Dorothy*

Sometimes Dad forgot he ate and wanted to eat again. I kept small containers of applesauce or a couple of cookies on hand. I couldn't let him gain too much weight or I wouldn't have been able to lift him. — *Marie*

If your family enjoyed going out to eat on a regular basis, continue doing it for as long as possible. The goal is to keep your parent engaged in normal activities as long as possible. If your parent shows signs of agitation at a restaurant, it may be due to excessive noise or strange surroundings. Try finding a quieter, more relaxed restaurant the next time and see if that helps. If it doesn't, it may be time to have all meals at home. — *Shirley*

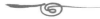

Driving

Driving, and the ability of your parent to continue driving, is a common concern for caregivers. Driving demands constant split-second decisions and reactions as well as good judgment — all of which are seriously compromised with Alzheimer's. Restricting (or eliminating) your parent's driving privileges can be excruciatingly difficult since it means further restrictions to their independence.

Your family may have already discussed — or have a plan in place — to determine when the time is right to restrict or take away your parent's driving privileges. If you don't, or if you are having difficulty deciding if it is still safe for your parent to be behind the wheel, begin by taking a short drive (down the street or around the block) with your parent. On the drive, watch for the following:

- ❑ Failure to obey traffic signs or signals, such as traffic lights and stop signs.
- ❑ Failure to put on their seat belt.
- ❑ Driving too slow or too fast.
- ❑ Stopping at a green light and/or failure to stop at a red light.
- ❑ Inability or failure to yield.
- ❑ Getting lost or confused over which direction to turn at a crossroads.

❑ Difficulty judging distance of other vehicles.

❑ Becoming angry, hostile or confused while driving.

❑ Difficulty judging distance from curb or barriers or inability to stay within their lane.

❑ Confusing the brake and gas pedal.

❑ Seemingly oblivious to other cars or bicycles and/or pedestrians on the side of the road.

❑ Failure to check mirrors or blind spots when changing lanes or backing up.

Remember, we are looking for a *pattern* of behavior. If something happens once or twice, and never happens again, there may not be cause for concern. However, if things are happening more frequently, there is probably cause for concern and you may want to consider restricting, or taking away, your parent's driving privileges.

If you don't live close enough to your parent to personally do this, ask a neighbor, friend, or family member who lives nearby to ride with your parent. As we discussed in the prior chapter, listen and watch for things your parent says or does. For example, your parent may say "I had the silliest thing happen today. I got lost on my way home from the store." Or you may notice it is taking your parent much longer than normal to arrive home from a destination, indicating they may have gotten lost and were driving around trying to find their way home.

How to Stop Your Parent From Driving

Loss of driving privileges means loss of independence which can be upsetting or embarrassing to your parent. They may refuse to surrender their keys or license or try to sneak out and drive. Caregivers took a variety of steps to ensure their parent didn't harm themselves, or anyone else, by getting behind the wheel of a car. Here is what they suggest:

❑ Disable your parent's vehicle (disconnect the battery, remove the distributor cap or wires).

❑ Take away (or hide) their keys.

❑ Hide or sell their car. Out of sight, out of mind.

❑ Check your state's driving regulations. Some states require physicians to report a diagnosis of Alzheimer's to the state health department who, in turn, is required to report it to the Department of Motor Vehicles (DMV). The DMV then has the right to re-test the individual, recommend a safe driving course or revoke their driver's license.

❑ Some caregivers notified their local law enforcement and encouraged them to stop their parent if they saw them driving and issue a citation.

❑ Talk with your parent's physician about your concerns. He or she may want to check for any physical or visual problems that may be causing your parent's driving difficulties.

❑ If the doctor rules out any physical or visual problems, he or she may be able to talk to your parent and convince them to stop driving. They may respond to hearing it from a trusted professional, rather than you. Alternatively, since your parent may also be likely to follow a doctor's orders, the doctor may be able to write a "Do Not Drive" prescription/order.

❑ Talk with your parent. Part of your parent's resistance may be concern that they won't be able to do the things they've always done. If that's your parent's concern, put a plan in place to address those concerns. Reach out to neighbors, friends and family who can drive your parent to the store, doctor's office or other appointments. Arrange for friends to stop by on a regular basis to visit your parent. Keep the names and phone numbers of people who are willing to drive your parent (as well as contact information for any local taxi or community transportation services) readily available.

❑ Before providing your parent with the name and number of a taxi or transportation, consider contacting the company and advising them of your parent's condition. You may ask that they contact you before picking up your parent to ensure your parent doesn't get lost or wander too far from home.

❑ You may also get guidance or assistance with this problem from a variety of local or national organizations or professionals (law enforcement, senior groups, AAA, AARP, etc.)

❑ Build and maintain a social network for your parent so they don't feel isolated.

❑ Consider home-delivery of medication, groceries and meals to further reduce the necessity of driving.

I started doing all the driving so Dad got out of the habit of driving. — *Allyson*

I didn't want to be the one to tell Mom she couldn't drive so I asked her doctor to write her a letter stating she shouldn't drive or live alone until she was healthy again. We also disabled her van after we heard she was out driving after dark and had stopped on the freeway. — *Bonnie*

You'll know when it's time for your parent to stop driving. When it came time for Mom to stop, we took both sets of car keys and told her we couldn't find them even though we acted like we were helping her search for them. We also kept her car at my brother's house and, after a while, she stopped asking about it. I think she enjoyed us taking her wherever she needed to go because it took the pressure off of her. — *Dorothy*

Dad would ask me for the car keys but I just never seemed to have them. — *Marie*

Last week I caved in and let Dad drive my daughter and me three blocks to the beach. He ran a stop sign 100 feet from the house and nearly drove us into oncoming traffic. He believes he stopped at the sign and there is no point in telling him otherwise. He won't believe it and it will just upset him. I made sure I told my mother and siblings what happened but I'm alone in this battle. No one will help me get him to stop driving and I don't know what to do. My parents act like I'm the enemy but I live in eternal fear that he'll kill or maim someone's child by getting behind the wheel. — *Pam*

If you wouldn't put your child or grandchild in the car with them, it's time to have the difficult discussion about driving. — *Rhonda*

PART TWO: Behavioral Problems

As the disease progresses, your parent may begin to exhibit difficult or uncharacteristic behaviors which include wandering, pacing, irritability, sleep problems, hallucinations or delusions, verbal or physical aggression, violence, and inappropriate behavior.

Most of the time, your parent's disruptive or disturbing behavior doesn't just happen. It is often triggered by something that has happened or something someone said or did. It could also be caused by a change of circumstances or environment, fatigue, overstimulation, a change in activity level, or the feeling they are losing control or having control taken away from them. It could also be caused (or escalated) by an underlying medical problem or drug interaction.

Find The Trigger

Since your parent can't communicate what is causing them distress it is up to you, as their caregiver, to try and determine the cause — or trigger — behind their behavior. Finding and removing the triggers and changing, or adapting, their environment may eliminate or lessen the chance of the problematic behavior from occurring or recurring.

Begin by ruling out any possible underlying medical conditions or possible drug interaction. Many caregivers report that increased agitation or behavioral problems were often a fairly accurate indicator of the presence of a urinary tract infection (UTI). This is not to say any and all agitated behavior is the result of a UTI — however, it is worth considering and ruling out.

Your parent may not be feeling well due to another chronic illness or health problem they have, such as diabetes or constipation. Impaired vision or hearing can add to your parent's confusion so you may consider getting their hearing or vision checked. Individuals with Alzheimer's or dementia are particularly vulnerable to the side effects of medication, combining medications or overmedication (especially if your parent is handling their own medication). Medication can cause drowsiness, confusion, agitation, increased thirst or dryness of the mouth. Report any possible side effects to your parent's doctor immediately.

Watch Your Parent's Behavior

Once you've ruled out a medical problem or drug interaction, begin looking for other possible causes for their behavior. If you recently changed your parent's caregiving or living arrangements, they may be tired or confused by the new activities or people in their daily life. New places, spaces and faces can trigger disruptive or troubling behavior. If your parent is tugging or pulling at their clothing it may indicate they need to use the bathroom.

Caregivers say by watching your parent's behavior you may be able to determine the cause and address it immediately. Consider if your parent may be feeling:

- Rushed? Slow down.
- Confused? Break the task into small, easily-understood steps.
- Bored? Find ways to involve your parent in what you are doing or give your parent a small task to keep them busy and allow them to feel needed.
- Tired, overtired or fatigued? Stop what you're doing and allow your parent to rest.
- Agitated? Perhaps there's too much noise or stimulation. Go to a quieter place where there are fewer people or things to stimulate them.
- A lack of control? Sometimes allowing your parent to do things for themselves restores a sense of control and helps calm down disruptive behavior.

Watch Your Behavior

Your behavior, and how you act, react, and handle any given situation with your parent, can have a direct, and dramatic, impact on your parent's behavior and the end result. Here's what our caregivers recommend:

❑ Don't confront, argue with, or criticize your parent.

❑ Acknowledge your parent's frustration.

❑ Remain calm and positive.

❑ Speak slowly and quietly.

❑ Be understanding and reassure your parent that he (or she) is safe.

❑ Try diversionary tactics (go for a walk, redirect them to another activity or place, or try to distract them).

❑ Slow down and create, restore or maintain a calm atmosphere.

❑ If necessary, move to a quieter or calmer location.

❑ Don't take things personally.

❑ Keep your sense of humor.

❑ Be flexible.

❑ Be creative.

❑ Talk to others and find out what worked for them.

Mom was the sweetest person on earth but her personality went through many changes with Alzheimer's. At times, she would fly off the handle for no reason. When she did, we just put our arms around her and talked to her in a really soothing voice. She would always calm down. We never had to medicate her for agitation. Love goes a long way. — **Dorothy**

Adjust the Environment

Sometimes making a small adjustment to your parent's environment can have a huge impact on their behavior.

❑ Reduce or eliminate any loud, disturbing noise.

❑ Turn off violent or fast-paced television shows. Instead, turn on comedies, children's cartoons or shows that will relax and calm your parent.

❑ Distract them with an activity (go for a walk, look at photos together, or just sit and talk).

❑ Limit or restrict the number of people in the room to reduce noise, confusion or overstimulation.

❑ Sometimes your parent's environment can make it difficult for them to hear, see or use their senses. Again, look at the environment through your *parent's* eyes and make adjustments to lighting or sound as necessary.

❑ New or unfamiliar places can be upsetting or make your parent feel lost, confused or abandoned. Reassure your parent and return to a safe, familiar environment.

PART THREE: Specific Behavioral Problems

In the following section, we'll discuss individual behaviors. While many of the adjustments, modifications and responses we just discussed can be applied in these situations as well, caregivers also shared suggestions or remedies specific to these behaviors. We'll begin by addressing a behavior that was a major concern for many caregivers: wandering.

Wandering

Statistics show that six out of every ten individuals with Alzheimer's will wander and, if they aren't found within 24 hours, they risk serious injury or death. Therefore, wandering — or just the thought of wandering — is terrifying to most caregivers.

Caregivers say wandering usually didn't happen without reason or warning. They say the key to reducing, or eliminating, the possibility of your parent wandering is to try and determine what might be causing the behavior.

Some caregivers say wandering doesn't necessarily mean leaving home but can also mean wandering around *inside* the home, disoriented and unable to find their way from one spot to the next. However, I'd like to clarify that *in this book*, that type of behavior would be considered pacing. What we are talking about in this section is wandering outside — *and away from* — the home.

There are two basic types of wandering. Being aware of the type of wandering your parent seems susceptible to may assist you in figuring out how to address the problem. The first is when your parent wanders for a purpose or reason — even if it is unrealistic. For example, your parent may wander because they believe they're going to work, or going to feed the chickens, or going home. With this type of wandering it is as if your parent is repeating a behavior from their past.

The other type of wandering is when your parent appears to be wandering aimlessly or without a specific purpose. This type of wandering may be an attempt by your parent to get re-oriented to their surroundings or the situation.

Caregivers say, in hindsight, there were behaviors or "red flags" in advance of their parent's wandering but they either hadn't paid attention or didn't realize the behavior could lead to wandering. Those behaviors included:

- an inability to recognize familiar people or surroundings.
- looking for someone (especially a deceased family member, friend or pet).
- increased restlessness.
- increased requests to "go home" (even if their parent was already in theirs home).

Many caregivers feel that wandering, like many other behaviors associated with Alzheimer's, is their parent's attempt to communicate. They say it's important to try and determine, through their behavior, what your parent is trying to tell you. Are they hungry, tired, or confused? Are they bored? Is there something that may have triggered a memory of something outside? Has their doctor recently changed their medication? Are they in a new, confusing or upsetting situation or environment?

Caregivers suggest the following:

❑ Regular exercise or activity can minimize restlessness. Caregivers say having their parent involved in an adult day center or other activity where they were regularly stimulated (physically and mentally) helped eliminate any desire to wander.

❑ Take your parent for a walk. Exercise can help reduce agitation that can lead to wandering.

❑ Be careful not to overtire or over-stimulate your parent since caregivers say it can trigger a desire to wander.

❑ Give your parent a small task or chore to do. One woman kept a basket of towels in the closet so that when her father grew restless and wanted to leave the house, she'd pull out the basket and ask him to fold the towels. Her father wasn't aware he was folding the same towels over and over again but it didn't matter. He felt needed and it kept him busy, happy and safe in the house.

❑ Provide your parent with a snack or something to drink.

❑ Remind your parent to go — or take them — to the bathroom.

❑ Reduce any excessive noise or sounds. Try to create, or restore, a calm, quiet environment for your parent.

❑ Watch to see if your parent's restlessness or desire to wander happens at a regular time of day.

My mother tried to leave the house around the same time every day to "feed the chickens." Initially, I thought it was simply a memory of something she'd done as a little girl on the farm. However, one day I saw my mother looking out the window and watching our neighbor walk her dog. Mom immediately wanted to leave the house to go "feed the chickens." I realized Mom's desire to go outside was being triggered by seeing the neighbor walk her dog so I began planning activities at that time of day that kept Mom away from the window and her desire to leave to go "feed the chickens" vanished. —Jaye

There are also things you can do within your home to discourage wandering and keep your parent safe and secure.

❑ Help your parent find their way around the house by putting pictures on interior doors to serve as visual cues. One caregiver bought a "Restroom" sign for the bathroom door at an office supply store. As soon as she put it up, her father stopped wandering. Apparently, her father, in an attempt to find the bathroom, had been opening the front door and walking out.

- ❑ Use nightlights and make sure the house is well lit, especially at night, to avoid the possibility of your parent getting lost and wandering outside.
- ❑ Disguise outside exits and doors. Hang a curtain over them. Paint, wallpaper or put a mural on the door to make it "fade" into the background.
- ❑ Put a stop sign on doors leading outside.
- ❑ Remove any visual cues or triggers which might remind your parent of leaving the house. Remove key or shoe racks near the door. If your parent takes their glasses or purse with them when they leave, make sure they aren't kept in the vicinity of the front door.
- ❑ Place solid black mats in front of doors leading to the outside. For individuals with Alzheimer's, these can appear as deep holes and may keep your parent from wandering.
- ❑ Install alarms on doors and windows — and motion detectors outside the home.
- ❑ Consider using floor mats and/or bed pads with built-in remote alarms to alert you if your parent gets out of bed at night. Some caregivers use baby monitors (or similar devices).
- ❑ Install a security system both inside and outside your home.
- ❑ Create a "safe area" where your parent can garden, sit or be outdoors without the possibility of wandering away.

If Your Parent Wanders: Ensuring Their Safe Return

Regardless of how diligent you are about watching your parent, they may still get out of the house and wander away. Therefore, it's imperative to do everything possible to ensure that, if your parent does wander away, they are returned quickly and safely. This includes:

❑ Having your parent wear an ID bracelet, necklace or other form of identification at all times.

❑ Putting your parent's name and emergency phone numbers on every piece of clothing, either with tags or by writing it on their clothing with a permanent fabric marker.

❑ Placing ID cards inside your parent's wallet or purse.

One of our caregivers prepared a flier which she gave to friends, family, neighbors, and local law enforcement and emergency personnel. The flier included:

❑ A recent photo of her parent.

❑ Information on her parent (including height, weight and any easily-identifiable behaviors or marks) as well as the fact that he is in excellent physical condition and can walk quickly.

❑ An explanation that her parent has Alzheimer's and that attempts at approaching or confronting him directly might add to his confusion. Therefore, the flier suggests immediately notifying family and/or local law enforcement.

❑ Contact information for every family member or contact (including cell and home phone numbers) as well as the number for local law enforcement and emergency personnel.

❑ Any time there was any change in her father's condition, living arrangements or contact information, she updated the flier, retrieved the old ones and provided everyone with copies of the new flier.

❑ Some caregivers use a GPS system. With an ever-increasing number of GPS systems available, you may want to ask others to see what has worked for them but choose a system that will work for you, your parent and your specific set of circumstances.

❑ Caregivers suggest enrolling your parent in either a national or local program that would help ensure their safe return. Many communities and municipalities are involved with Project Lifesaver International (PLI), which provides response to families of adults who might wander due to Alzheimer's or dementia. The Alzheimer's Association also has a Safe Return Program available. See the *Resource* section for contact information on these programs.

❏ If your parent is (or will be) moving to a different location — either now or in the future — find out what programs are available in the new location and register your parent in advance of the move.

- Enrolling your parent in a full-time day care will keep your parent busy and safe and limit opportunities for them to wander. — *Allyson*

- Wandering became such a problem that the home health care nurse told us to get a home monitor. Gratefully, my mother only tried to wander during the day. — *Dorothy*

- Keep up-to-date photos or videos of your loved one readily available. Even if your parent has never wandered, be prepared for the possibility and take precautionary measures. — *Frank*

- I kept plastic dishes in the sink and Dad would wash them over and over again. I also kept a basket of towels for him to fold over and over again. — *Marie*

- The only jewelry Mom ever wore consistently was a watch. I knew she'd never wear an ID necklace or bracelet, so I bought her a medic alert watch and had her name, my cell phone number and "Alzheimer's" engraved on the back of the watch. She wore it every day. — *Patti*

- Emergency personnel should know how to contact all family members — not just the primary caregiver. — *Shirley*

Sundowning

For some caregivers, the late afternoon and evening is the most difficult time of the day. After a long day of caring for your parent, and just as your energy and patience may be wearing thin, you parent's behavior may worsen. They may become irritable, agitated, fearful, disoriented or restless. Many call this behavior "sundowning" (a reference to the fact that it occurs later in the day when the sun goes down).

Theories about why sundowning occurs range from fatigue and a diminished capacity to handle stress to increased confusion caused by darkness or shadows. Other possibilities include: medication, illness, pain, drinking too much caffeine or alcohol, eating too many stimulating foods, overstimulation, the room or environment being too hot (or cold), or sleeping too much during the day.

Caregivers say the following was helpful:

- ❏ Schedule your day and activities to address the problem. Plan any physical or stimulating activities for early in the day. Late afternoon and evening hours should be quiet and calm so plan structured, quiet activities (listening to music, playing a simple card game, or going for a short walk) for later in the day.

- ❏ Try giving your parent a healthy snack (like fruit or yogurt) in the afternoon to avoid a late afternoon energy slump.

- ❏ Eliminate (or reduce) stimulating foods (such as sugar, caffeine, caffeinated drinks and junk food) from your parent's diet. If you're unable to completely eliminate these foods, try giving them early in the day so the effects wear off by bedtime. Caffeine alone can stay in the system for up to eight hours. Also be aware that "decaffeinated" drinks often still contain some level of caffeine so, instead, look for "caffeine-free" drinks and beverages.

- ❏ Before bed, consider giving your parent a light snack or a cup of herbal tea or warm milk.

- ❏ Close the curtains and adjust the lighting before dusk to help minimize shadows and darkness.

- ❏ Develop and try to maintain a bedtime routine. Try to have your parent go to bed at the same time every night.

- ❏ If your parent wanders at night, check, and double-check, to ensure your home is safe. Put anything that could be a potential danger out of sight or reach of your parent. Keep a nightlight on in hallways, bathrooms and their bedroom. Lock doors and block off stairs.

❏ Make sure your parent is getting enough exercise during the day and consider increasing their level of activity. However, be aware of the fine line between too much and not enough activity. You want your parent to be busy enough during the day so they're tired at bedtime but, if they've been kept too busy, they may get overtired or agitated and find it difficult (or impossible) to sleep.

❏ Try getting your parent up earlier or keeping them up later at night to discourage them from spending too much time in bed.

❏ Discourage long naps during the day.

❏ If your parent refuses to go to bed, allow them to sleep on the couch or in a reclining chair.

❏ If you, or any of your parent's caregivers, aren't getting enough sleep, consider asking a friend or family member (or hiring someone) to come in to allow you to get a good night's sleep. If you can't find someone to come for an entire evening, perhaps you can find someone to relieve you for a few hours during the day so you can take a catnap. Any sleep is better than no sleep. You need to maintain and preserve your health and energy so you can properly care for your loved one.

❏ Be extremely cautious about the use of sleep medication — whether over-the-counter or prescription medication — for you or your parent. These can sometimes have the opposite effect (or interact with other medication) and create new problems.

• I tried to visit Mom in the late afternoon or early evening. We'd go for a walk or just sit and talk. It seemed to minimize her pacing and helped with sundowning. — *Ann*

• Mom worried any time we went out because she thought it was absolutely necessary to be back home, in her familiar environment, before it got dark. We could sense when she was getting nervous and would reassure her. If the sun went down before we could get her home, she'd stay overnight with one of us. — *Dorothy*

• One day, I pulled Mom's old rocking chair out of storage and, in doing so, finally found something that helped with her sun-downing. I don't know if it was because she was physically exhausted but unable to settle herself mentally but the chair allowed her to sit and relax while also keeping her "busy." Maybe it brought back old memories. Whatever it was, I didn't care. I was just happy we'd found something that helped. — *Jaye*

• In the late afternoon and evening, Dad would get antsy and wander or get upset about going home — even though he was already in his home. I paid attention to when it would begin and, before it got out of control, I kept him busy doing puzzles or playing cards. — *Marie*

Repetitive Questions

Answering the same question over and over, or hearing the same story a hundred times over the course of one day, while harmless, can be stressful to a caregiver. Sometimes repetitive questions can be an indication that your parent is bored or anxious about something. Try distracting them with a new activity or snack. Some caregivers suggest ignoring the behavior or question while other caregivers say ignoring it only made the situation worse. Find, and do, what works with your parent.

Repetitive questions or repeatedly telling the same story over and over, like so many behaviors that accompany Alzheimer's, will disappear over time.

Pacing, Agitation and Fear

Pacing, agitation, nervousness, anxiety and fear occur for a number of reasons. It may be changes occurring in your parent's brain, a natural reaction to constantly feeling lost or confused, or feeling tense or troubled by something that is happening.

Individuals with Alzheimer's can be extremely sensitive to the mood and general "vibe" of the people and space around them. You may think you're hiding your concerns or fears (or the argument you and your husband had this morning) from your parent but, many times, they will pick up on things and act or react in response to what they are sensing.

Our caregivers recommend the following when dealing with pacing, agitation, or fear:

- ❑ Remain calm and talk to your parent in a calm, quiet manner.
- ❑ Adjust the environment, as necessary, to restore calm and quiet.
- ❑ Avoid caffeinated beverages, sugar and "junk" food from your parent's diet.
- ❑ Reassure your parent with a hug or a touch.
- ❑ If your parent is fidgeting, pacing or restless, give them something to do or take them for a walk.
- ❑ Be aware of the general mood and atmosphere in the home. If you, or another family member, is tense or agitated consider stepping away from the situation and calming down.
- ❑ Don't argue with your parent. Even if their fear has no basis in reality, to them it is very real.

- This was a problem. She would get very agitated when she didn't know where my dad was so we got a white board and wrote messages for her to serve as reminders (e.g. "Daddy is up in his office" or "Daddy is outside"). It helped calm her down. — *Janice*
- Keeping things quiet helps a lot — *Jeannot*

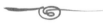

Hiding, Hoarding or Losing Items

Many individuals with Alzheimer's begin hiding and hoarding items. Others put things down, or move them to a different location and then forget where they put them. The result is the same: your keys, jewelry or money are missing.

Avoid asking your parent where the item is. They won't remember. Don't chastise or accuse your parent of stealing, losing or hiding the item, as this may only escalate the problem. Instead, caregivers suggest the following:

- ❑ Move (or remove) any valuables to a safe, secure location inaccessible by your parent.

- ❑ If hiding or hoarding money is the problem, try giving your parent small amounts of money they can keep in their pocket or handbag. Some caregivers gave their parent fake/play money which satisfied their parent's desire to still have money.

- ❑ If your parent suspects their money, or other object, is missing (and you know it's not) help them look for it. Then slowly direct them to where the "missing" item is or distract them towards another activity.

- ❑ Play detective and try to find your parent's favorite hiding place(s) or, better yet, limit the number of available hiding place(s) by locking closets or drawers.

Delusions and Hallucinations

Delusions and hallucinations are two different behaviors and it's important a caregiver be able to distinguish between the two.

Delusions are false beliefs your parent thinks are real (such as the belief that someone is trying to kill them or that their husband isn't really their spouse). Delusions may result from your parent misinterpreting a situation.

Hallucinations, on the other hand, are sensory in nature and can involve any of the senses: sight, smell, taste, touch, and hearing. Your parent may see or hear things that others don't, that can't be verified by anyone else, or that don't exist. They may have conversations with people who aren't there or see insects crawling up the wall.

Both behaviors can be distressing to a caregiver. To see your once loving and trusting parent suddenly turn paranoid, suspicious, jealous, or accusatory towards you or another family member can be very upsetting. It's important that you don't take it personally. No matter what your parent accuses you or another family member of, it's important to remember it is part of the disease.

Caregivers suggest, when dealing with your parent's delusions or hallucinations, to:

- ❑ Avoid disagreeing or arguing with your parent. While their accusations or what they are seeing, hearing or believing may seem ludicrous to you, to them it is very real. Arguing or disagreeing with them, or trying to convince them they're wrong, usually only makes the situation worse.
- ❑ Try to remain calm, reassure your parent and try to distract them.
- ❑ Keep rooms well-lit to lessen shadows.
- ❑ Check for glare or reflections on windows, floors, walls or furniture.
- ❑ Close all blinds, curtains and drapes before dark.
- ❑ Ask your parent to point to what they are seeing or hearing. It may be that they are seeing their reflection on the TV screen or window and simply no longer recognize their face.

For some caregivers, unless the hallucination was causing severe or aggressive behavior, they weren't overly concerned and chose to ignore it. If the hallucination isn't dangerous or upsetting to your parent, determine if there is anything you really *need* to do. Perhaps it's more upsetting to you than your parent that they are seeing or having conversations with their deceased mother. Some caregivers wondered if the truth was their parent was simply able to see things they couldn't.

If your parent is having increased incidents, or you are getting increasingly concerned, talk with your parent's doctor to make sure there isn't a possible underlying physical or mental condition (such as a side effect of medication, poor eyesight or hearing, or an underlying illness, pain or infection). Also consider having your parent's eyesight or hearing checked (or, at the very least, make sure they are wearing their glasses and/or hearing aid).

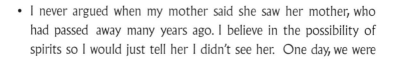

- • I never argued when my mother said she saw her mother, who had passed away many years ago. I believe in the possibility of spirits so I would just tell her I didn't see her. One day, we were visiting Mom and we noticed a leaf from her kitchen table leaning against the basement door. When I asked her why it was there she said it was to keep the people from coming up out of the basement into her kitchen. We left it there because, if nothing else, it made her feel better. — *Bonnie*

- About 6–8 months before she passed, my grandmother began having hallucinations that there were bugs constantly crawling on the walls. I believe those were a side effect of her medication. But there were other hallucinations, where she'd stare off into a corner and kind of smile or appear deep in thought. When I asked her what she was staring at, she would turn to me with a blank expression. She never had an answer. I have no idea what she saw — whether it was a hallucination or just something I couldn't see. — *Cassie*

- We mixed up lavender essential oil in a spray bottle for my father. Every time Dad saw something that frightened him, we'd hand him the bottle and he'd start spraying whatever it was he saw. I think this helped give him some control over what he was seeing and since the scent of lavender is relaxing it made the room smell wonderful and also helped calm everyone down. — *Frank*

- I kept in mind what someone once told me: that to someone with Alzheimer's the hallucinations are very real and to think how terrified or upset I would be if I were seeing things and other people were telling me they weren't real. — *Leslie*

- Hallucination? What hallucination? Who's to say my grandmother or my mother's sister weren't in the room with Mom? Maybe it wasn't a hallucination. Maybe the problem was that they were really there but I just wasn't able to see them. — *Patti*

- Look for the trigger, or source, of the hallucination. Did your parent pass by a window or mirror and see their reflection? Has your parent developed an illness? My father had terrible hallucinations whenever he was developing (or had) a urinary tract infection — and the hallucinations were worse when he was placed on antibiotics to combat the infection. — *Shirley*

Inappropriate Behavior

As the disease progresses, your parent's filters regarding what is appropriate or acceptable behavior disappears. They may say or do something inappropriate or completely out-of-character. One caregiver said her quiet, demure, ladylike mother was now cursing like a drunken sailor; another that his normally reserved, modest father was constantly trying to take off his clothes in public.

How you act and react to inappropriate behavior is important. Remain calm and try to redirect your parent (or their attention) elsewhere. If they are attempting to remove their clothing (or already have), tell them their behavior is not appropriate and quietly and calmly help them refasten or put their clothing back on.

Some caregivers were concerned because their parent was exhibiting signs of sexually inappropriate behavior in public or inappropriately touching themselves or someone else. One caregiver was fearful her father's behavior could possibly become a danger to himself or others. If you have ongoing, or growing, concerns about your parent's inappropriate or irrational behavior, talk with your parent's doctor or other healthcare professional for advice.

- I recall one minor episode while out shopping for bras with my mother. Since she had lost so much weight, I couldn't go by her old bras and had no idea what size to buy her. Sensing my confusion, Mom lifted up her shirt and showed me her breasts. I gently pulled her shirt back down, gave her a hug, and thanked her for her help. My mother was one of the most modest women I knew and normally would have never done such a thing. However, in her current mental state, she thought she was simply being helpful. — *Jaye*

- After a while, I thought of Dad like a child. When he did something inappropriate, I reminded myself it was just the disease. — *Marie*

- Mom always loved going to church, so one Mother's Day my dad and I took Mom to church. The priest had a thick accent and it was difficult to understand what he was saying. He was also extremely long-winded. At one point during the sermon, the priest paused to take a breath. The church was absolutely silent and Mom, in a very loud and distinct voice, said, "Jesus Christ! Is he <u>ever</u> gonna shut up?" People around us chuckled and the priest ended the sermon not too long after Mom's comment. I believe there's a Bible verse for moments like that — and so many others — with our parent and Alzheimer's: "Forgive them, for they know not what they do." — *Patti*

Aggression or Violence

Aggression may be physical (your parent hits or shoves you) or verbal (they shout, scream or call you names) and can occur suddenly and for no apparent reason. Other times, there is an environmental or physical reason behind the behavior.

- Your parent may be overtired or overstimulated.
- Your parent's doctor recently changed their medication.
- Your parent is in pain or has an infection or other physical ailment.
- Your parent feels lost, confused, or overwhelmed.
- There's too much noise or too many people in your parent's immediate environment.

Caregivers suggest the following:

- ❑ Try to remain calm and find the cause behind your parent's behavior. Think about what happened — or what was said — just prior to their aggression.
- ❑ Remove, or limit, noise or distractions.
- ❑ Remove your parent from the environment or situation.
- ❑ Don't argue or get angry or upset with your parent.
- ❑ Try to distract them and steer them (and their focus) to another activity.
- ❑ Turn on relaxing music.

When responding to aggressive behavior, it's important that first — and foremost — you assess the situation and any immediate danger to your parent, yourself or anyone else. If you believe that you, or anyone else, is in imminent danger, it's important to leave or remove yourself from the scene. Stand out of direct reach of your parent and call for help — a neighbor, family member, friend or doctor — or call 911 and/or your local police or emergency personnel. Don't try to physically restrain your parent, unless it is absolutely necessary, as this can often make the situation worse.

PART FOUR: Diversionary Tactics

Diversionary tactics are things you can do to help diffuse or steer your parent away from a stressful, unsafe, difficult or potentially volatile situation. We've already discussed a number of diversionary tactics — from remaining calm to distracting your parent. In this section, we're going to discuss a few additional diversionary techniques: staying active with your parent, music, touch, and animals. Each of these, whether used alone or in combination with other diversionary tactics, can help manage, decrease or prevent difficult or unpleasant behaviors and also contribute to your parent's quality of life.

Keeping Your Parent Active

Continuing to integrate your parent into everyday life by keeping them with (and around) other people and places can help stimulate them physically and mentally. However, one of the challenges caregivers face is finding appropriate activities for your parent — and constantly reassessing and changing those activities as your parent's abilities and skill levels shift.

Begin by considering what kind of activities your parent enjoyed doing *before* Alzheimer's. If they liked to dance, put on some music and dance! If they enjoyed shopping, go to a mall and window shop. If your mother enjoyed knitting, while she may no longer be able to knit, she may enjoy rolling up balls of yarn. If your father drew or painted, give him crayons and coloring books. If your parent was very social, consider an adult day program or inviting friends or family to visit.

Caregivers suggest, and had success with, the following activities:

- **Walking.** Even short walks can provide exercise and keep your parent's joints moving, their muscles healthy and may even help them get a better night's sleep. Make sure your parent is dressed appropriately for the weather and conditions (including comfortable, supportive footwear). Before engaging in any physical exercise or activity, talk to your parent's doctor. There may be limitations you aren't aware of and the doctor may also be able to guide you towards activities that are appropriate for your parent.

- **Playing games.** Playing childhood games — or simple adaptations of those games — can provide ongoing entertainment and relaxation. Caregivers say dominoes, Yahtzee, bowling, jigsaw puzzles or simple card games are some of their parent's favorites.

- **Adult day programs.** Many caregivers say the routine, socialization and planned activities provided by an adult day program made a huge difference in their parent's mood, memory and sleep patterns.

Dan Koffman's father was diagnosed with dementia in the early 1980s and his mother was the primary caregiver. An artist who believed in the simple truth that "a picture is worth a thousand words," Koffman designed a picture book series — first for his father and eventually for others with Alzheimer's and dementia (individuals Koffman calls "Special Seniors").

Simple Pleasures for Special Seniors is a series of books filled with simple, bold photo illustrations of objects and aspects of life easily recognized by most Special Seniors. The first three books in the series are *Fruits, Fun Foods* and *Hand Tools.*

"My dad was a tool guy. He was always in his workshop building or fixing something," Koffman said. "When he looked through the *Tools* book, he told us stories that made my mother smile and gave the whole family moments of joy and something precious to remember."

"I wanted to do something that would have a positive effect on people suffering from dementia as well as those who love and care for them," he said. "*Simple Pleasures for Special Seniors* is the realization of that goal."

Planning Activities and Outings

Caregivers say taking your parent out in public can be relaxing and rewarding for you and your parent — or it can be terribly disruptive and upsetting. Much depends on your parent's mood, your mood, where you go, and the environment.

Some caregivers say taking their parent to a quiet restaurant was better than taking them to a family restaurant where there was a lot of noise and children running around. Others say the family restaurant was better because their parent loved watching the children laugh and play. Again, it comes down to being sensitive (and aware) of your parent's mood and what brings them joy — and what agitates them.

Plan activities and outings at a time of day when your parent is typically the least agitated and most agreeable. However, once you've made your plans, remain flexible. If you have something planned and your parent is having a particularly bad day, reschedule or cancel.

- Short time periods in a comfortable, known setting — like church or a family restaurant — seemed to lessen Mom's anxiety. — *Ann*

- Mom loved to go anywhere. She was a people watcher and loved to go out to shop and watch the other people. — *Bonnie*

- Be aware of the amount of noise and commotion when you eat out. Some people with Alzheimer's can't handle too much noise or activity. — *Jeannot*

- I had business cards that said: "This is my mother who I love very much. She has Alzheimer's. Thank you for your understanding and patience." I kept a supply of the cards with me at all times. If we were out in public and Mom got angry or difficult, I would give a card to whomever might be impacted or affected by her behavior — a waiter, store clerk, or someone seated in the waiting room with us. It eliminated the need for me to explain Mom's behavior in front of her (which could further escalate the problem). It also allowed the other person to understand the reason behind Mom's behavior. Some people thanked me for the explanation. Most people became more understanding and patient with my mother and sometimes followed my lead to try and calm Mom down. — *Patti*

• Some of the distress about going out in public may be your concern about what people will think if your parent does something outrageous. Be confident. Know you can handle the situation and that other people will respond according to how they see you handling the situation. If you are calm and poised, they'll follow your cue and respond with the same kind of firm, quiet poise. — *Shirley*

• We take Dad everywhere. We just know in advance that everything will take longer than it normally would and that he may get tired and want to leave. — *Wanda*

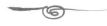

Car Rides

Many caregivers say their parent loved going for a ride in the car and that it often helped relax or calm their parent down. They also suggest:

❑ Have your parent use the bathroom before you venture out. If your parent is having bouts of incontinence, consider putting waterproof covers on your car seats.

❑ Bring along a snack and drink.

❑ If your parent needs it, help them put on and take off their seatbelt.

❑ Keep a travel bag in the car with wipes, a blanket, and change of clothes (including an extra pair of regular/disposable underwear).

❑ Don't ever leave your parent alone in the car — even for a minute. They may panic and not remember how to get out of the car or they may accidentally put the car into gear by mistake. Any number of things could happen.

I wanted Mom to feel as normal as possible so we'd go for car rides. Almost always, we'd end up at Mom's favorite ice cream place where I'd order her favorite — a pineapple sundae. Even when she couldn't feed herself any more, I'd sit in the back seat with Mom and feed her the pineapple sundae. — **Dorothy**

♡

Mom went through a particularly difficult phase where it was almost impossible to find things that would relax or calm her down — both during the day and at night. Several professionals suggested enrolling her at our local adult day center.

On the first day, my dad dropped Mom off. When he returned home, I could see the sadness, and defeat, in his eyes so the next day I dropped Mom off and returned home. A few hours later, my dad pulled up in a brand new car.

Gone was their big black Mercury Grand Marquis and in its place was a shiny new bright red VW Beetle. I knew Dad had done this for Mom more than himself. Back in the '70s, my parents had a VW Beetle and Mom always loved that car — and red was her favorite color.

Dad was nervous when we went to pick Mom up that afternoon but as soon as she saw the new car, she was like a little kid! She giggled and laughed and clapped her hands.

Mom never went back to the adult day center. Instead, anytime she got upset or agitated, my dad would take her out for a ride and she would magically, and almost instantly, calm down. Anytime their bright red VW Beetle pulled into my driveway, the first words out of my mother's mouth were always, "Isn't this a beautiful car? I love the color!" — **Patti**

The Magic of Music

We've all heard the saying "Music soothes the savage beast" and evidence shows that it can — and does. The general consensus of numerous studies conducted on Alzheimer's patients over the years is that music decreases agitation and improves behavior. More specifically, the studies have shown music to:

- Improve the patient's mood as evidenced by their smiling, dancing or clapping to the music.
- Calm the patient during times of aggression or frustration, even during the difficult afternoon and evening hours.
- Make the patient more cooperative during bathing.
- Increase the number of hours of productive, restful sleep.

In my work as a music therapist, I've found that music heals the soul, releases physical pain, and improves an individual's cognitive awareness and memory recall and quality of life.

Some of the most beautiful, heartfelt work I have been blessed to do is my work with Alzheimer's and dementia clients in assisted living facilities. Many of them had forgotten who or where they were and asked, repeatedly, to "go home."

I have one very special memory of a client I'll call Walt. I was told that Walt was a happy man who loved music but was often unfocused and stared endlessly at the ceiling. Attempts to redirect Walt's gaze back into the room often left him afraid and confused.

During my one hour group sessions, I had them sing songs to induce memory recall. In order to engage them physically, I also had them use handheld percussion instruments. At my first group session with Walt, I approached him and began gently touching his hand. As I began to rock his hand to the beat of the song, Walt smiled and exhaled.

At our second group session, Walt began singing and rocked his hand to the beat of the music. There was no panic but he repeatedly asked to "go home."

After the third session, and Walt's constant requests to "go home," I decided to attempt to address feelings of "going home" through music. I came to the session with an arsenal of songs about home. Walt recognized every song and began tapping his neighbor to motivate them to sing along. The socialization within the group became contagious. I began asking what home meant to each of them. Walt was the most talkative, telling stories about his childhood and teen years, his home and life with his (now deceased) wife. He also talked about his children (who still visit him) in a positive, nurturing tone. We all listened intently.

Afterwards, one of the nurses told me Walt had always refused to remember, let alone talk about, his past. However, the songs had sparked happy memories that had been dormant for a long time and, for a brief moment in time, enhanced Walt's quality of life.

Prior to that session, Walt usually needed a weekly reminder of who I was and why I was there. However, after that session, when Walt saw me he would say, "Oh! You're the music lady that brought me back home."

Rebecca Ciurczak is a musician and music therapist.

Most caregivers find music to be extremely helpful in relaxing or soothing their parent and offer the following tips:

- ❑ Choose soothing, relaxing music since loud, unruly music can be upsetting or disorienting to your parent.
- ❑ Play music that is familiar to your parent — childhood nursery rhymes or songs from their era — as they can sometimes trigger long-term memories.
- ❑ Give your parent a small drum or handheld instrument. Having them identify the beat of a song exercises their ability to concentrate.
- ❑ Clap or sing along to the song — or get up and dance with your parent.

- • Music was a powerful ally for us — especially on Mom's bad days. Putting on an Eddie Arnold or Patsy Kline album would calm her down; a polka record would get her up off her chair and dancing. Watching the Lawrence Welk Show together became our Saturday night ritual. After every song, when Lawrence Welk clapped and said "Thank-a You" to the guests on his show, Mom thought he was talking to her. She would do this adorable little curtsy towards the TV and say "And thank-a you." For Mom, and us, music was magic. — *Patti*

- Near the end, my father no longer walked or talked and was mostly unresponsive. One day, when I came to visit him, I found all the residents gathered together for music recreation. When the singer started singing songs from my Dad's era, he started singing along. They had placed a sheet with the words to the songs on my father's lap but he never once used the sheet. Not once. He knew the words from memory. Hearing Dad's voice and hearing him sing was something I thought I'd never hear again. — *Shirley*

The following story came from Janice, one of our caregivers. It is about her friend, Pat, who had cared for both of her parents for many years. After her father died, Pat moved her mother in with her on her farm. Here is what Janice had to say about Pat, her mother, and music.

When I visit New Jersey, I usually stay with Pat and her mother, Rose, who is 93. They have an extremely close relationship and it's always a joy to be with them.

Pat decided to hire a full-time live-in caregiver so she can go out and do what needs to be done on the farm. However, since there weren't enough bedrooms in the house for the caregiver and her mother, Pat moved her mother into her bedroom. Having her mother sleep in the same bed is often difficult for Pat since Rose wakes up multiple times during the night. Although she is sometimes exhausted, Pat loves having her mother with her.

The last time I stayed with Pat and Rose, I discovered they love to sing together. First, one of them will sing a line then the other sings the next line until, finally, they join together to finish the song. It is beautiful to watch them gaze into each other's eyes. It is also quite amazing because, in spite of Rose's dementia, they have found a special way to bond and communicate with each other.

When I contacted Pat to get her permission to share this story, she agreed, saying that music had become a very special connection between her and her mother. She also told me, "*The latest thing Mom does is call me when she's in the other room, by singing, 'I Love Patty in the springtime, I love Patty in the fall, but most of all I love Patty all the time!' This brings tears to my eyes. Mom is a special delight!*"

Pat's story, and the following one from Mary K., are beautiful examples of how music can be a way for caregivers to continue to communicate with their parent.

Dad was a Southern Baptist from Kentucky and, before Alzheimer's, loved to play the organ and sing hymns. After he went into an Alzheimer's facility, I would sing him some of his favorite songs and Dad would join in, harmonizing beautifully.

One Saturday, I asked the facility if I could pick Dad up the next morning and take him with me to church. They agreed so, the next morning, I picked him up. Even though he no longer knew my name, Dad was always happy to see me and I could still see, and feel, the love for me in his eyes.

As we drove to my church, about an hour away, Dad and I sang and talked like two best friends. I explained to him that people in my church had been praying for him for a very long time and that we were going to repay them for their prayers with a song.

*When we arrived at church, Dad and I sat in the front pew. After the preacher introduced us, I took Dad's hand and we stood up and faced the congregation. I told everyone that Dad and I were there to share his favorite hymn to thank them for all their prayers. I wasn't sure if Dad would sing along but I started singing "Amazing Grace" anyway. Dad immediately joined in and sang with me like he'd never sung before. He had forgotten so many words — but not the words to this beautiful hymn. There wasn't a dry eye in the church. We were all blessed that day. — **Mary K.**

The Impact — and Importance — of Touch

Human beings not only like, but need, to be touched. Studies in orphanages and with premature babies over the years show that infants deprived of human touch lose weight, become ill and can die. Premature babies who are held, touched or massaged cry less, have a more relaxed pulse and respiration rate and gain more weight than premature babies who aren't touched.

Before we go any further, I want to make one thing very clear. As a society, we have become increasingly concerned and cautious about touch between individuals. Therefore, I want to clarify that we are talking about healthy, normal, nurturing and non-sexual touching between you and your parent — hugging your parent, holding their hand, or lightly stroking their back, forearm or shoulder.

Some caregivers say they or their parent were initially uncomfortable with touch because, through the years, family members didn't hug or touch one another. However, many of those same individuals pushed through their initial discomfort and found touch to be one more way to calm or connect with their parent. In addition, many caregivers said as the disease progressed, their parent — who may have been uncomfortable initially — began to relax and enjoy it.

It's important to be sensitive to your parent. Make eye contact, call them by name and gently touch their hand, arm or shoulder. Continue if, and only if, your parent seems open to physical contact.

Touch can help bring your parent into present time and space and help them focus or refocus. Touch can help decrease your parent's agitation, pacing and repetitive questions or behaviors by relaxing and reassuring them and helping them feel less anxious. Massaging your parent's shoulders, back or temples can help relieve tension or irritability. A nurturing, loving touch can also help your parent's health since studies have shown that touch (especially therapeutic touch or massage) helps lower a person's blood pressure, slows their heart rate and eases breathing. And, finally, touch can be a way for you to communicate and convey your love, compassion and respect to your parent.

The Joy of Animals

A pet often brings joy and unconditional love into our lives. Science and research are increasingly being led to believe that interaction with, or the mere presence of, an animal or pet can also have a positive impact on a person's physical health, including helping to lower blood pressure and blood triglyceride levels, lowering stress levels and increasing survival following a heart attack.

Therapy Dogs International, Inc. conducted a two-year study to determine what, if any, benefit animals had on clients, residents, patients and staff at a number of care facilities. Their findings included, among other things, "increased socialization, verbalization, alertness, and positive mood alterations."[1]

Many facilities now include animal therapy as a regular, and welcome, addition to their activity program with Alzheimer's patients. Animals can assist with agitation and also increase a patient's socialization and connection to the world. Some patients are reluctant to talk to people but are completely open and willing to interact and communicate with an animal — perhaps because animals are patient, loving and completely non-judgmental.

Nestled in the Piedmont region of North Carolina, Kopper Top Life Learning Center is a non-profit organization that provides therapeutic horseback riding along with recreational, animal-assisted and horticulture therapy to individuals with or without disabilities. Deborah Meredith, the Executive Director of Kopper Top, spoke about how animals can impact an individual with Alzheimer's.

Part of my work with Kopper Top is as a recreation therapist. I often take dogs, cats, rabbits, horses, goats and even chickens to facilities that have Alzheimer's patients. Since many of these individuals grew up with animals, these visits often trigger childhood memories and they'll often begin talking about a beloved pet or life on the farm. To encourage these memories, I'll ask them specific questions about the pet or life on the farm: "What was your pet's name?" or "Did you ride a mule to the fields?"

Even if a person has forgotten their pet's name, their faces light up, they smile and continue to socialize and reminisce as they pet and caress the therapy animals.

One woman we visited didn't respond to anyone or anything — except for a black Rex rabbit named Snuggles. Her face would light up when she saw Snuggles and she would begin talking and singing to the rabbit. She loved having Snuggles sit on her lap for hours. Once the rabbit was removed, she returned to absolute silence.

Animals give us true unconditional love and affection. They can brighten your parent's day — and give you the opportunity to connect or talk with your parent in a whole new way.

Deborah Meredith is the Executive Director of Kopper Top Life Learning Center as well as a licensed recreation therapist and certified therapeutic recreation specialist.

If you are considering introducing an animal into your parent's life outside of a traditional animal therapy program, you need to keep several things in mind. Dogs, cats, rabbits, guinea pigs, fish and horses have all been used to help alleviate the loneliness and isolation often experienced by Alzheimer's patients but not all animals may be appropriate for interaction with your parent. The ideal animal should be calm, gentle and have absolutely no aggressive tendencies since your parent may no longer know how to appropriately interact with an animal.

And, just as not all animals are appropriate candidates, not all Alzheimer's patients (including, possibly, your parent) are good candidates for animal therapy. Even if your parent always loved animals, they may not react or interact with them as you might hope. Make sure that someone is always nearby to oversee the interaction between the animal and your parent and can intercede, if necessary.

One caregiver said her mother had always been terrified of dogs. The first time her mother saw a therapy dog come into the care facility where she was living, she got extremely agitated and frightened. The handler immediately took the dog to another part of the building and the staff posted a sign on her mother's door indicating therapy dogs were not welcome in her room. Dog owners and handlers honored the sign and stayed out of her room and the staff made sure her mother was in her room with the door closed when therapy dogs were in the building.

For others, animals remained a welcome and healing part of their parent's day and routine.

> *Animals have always been a source of security and pleasure for my father. Before Alzheimer's, at the end of Dad's workday, you'd find him sitting on a bale of hay surrounded by barn cats and strays that had wandered in. More often than not, he'd have a cat on his lap.*
>
> *My son and I had adopted a dog named Butter who would sit at Dad's feet for hours as Dad stroked her head. Every so often, Butter would look up into Dad's eyes. She never did that with anyone else. It was almost as if Butter could sense Dad's illness and felt the need to stay close and protect him.*
>
> *After Dad moved into a facility, his eyes would lose some of their fixed stare whenever the therapy animals visited — and especially if a dog rested its head in Dad's lap.*
>
> *One of the greatest gifts my father ever received was a soft stuffed cat from my aunt. Dad carried it everywhere and held it on his lap and stroked it for hours. Even the nurses understood and, if Dad got agitated, all they had to do was retrieve his cat and he would calm down. — Shirley*

The Grandchild's Journey

For many grandchildren, their grandparent is a treasured and integral part of their life. When that grandparent — who has been a source of love, warmth and support — begins to exhibit curious, or even frightening, behavior it can be confusing and upsetting for a grandchild.

Alzheimer's can impact grandchildren on a number of different levels. First, they watch the disease take its toll on their grandparent. If their parent is a caregiver, they also see the day-to-day reality of the disease. Their parent's attention and time, which may have been devoted to them, is now being devoted to their grandparent. The grandchild may feel abandoned, neglected or jealous of how the disease has robbed them of time with their parent, and then feel guilty for feeling that way.

How a grandchild accepts, and perceives, their grandparent and Alzheimer's both now and in the future will depend upon their age, their past (and current) relationship with their grandparent, and the support and information provided to them. How, and by whom, the information is presented to a grandchild can also have an impact on them.

You may think you don't need to talk with a grandchild about their grandparent's diagnosis — or that you'll talk with them after they begin to ask questions. However, regardless of their age, children are naturally inquisitive. They are also very sensitive to changes in their environment and, in particular, at home and with loved ones. You may think you're keeping the diagnosis a secret from the grandchildren but they may have already sensed that something is awry. Some grandchildren may even believe they are somehow responsible for your discomfort, sadness or silence. Therefore, it's important to take the time to talk with them — and the sooner, the better.

Before your talk, think about what you're going to say. Consider any possible questions or concerns the grandchild might have and how you would answer those concerns. Be open and honest but only tell them what is age-appropriate. For younger children, you may not want to use the term, or words, "Alzheimer's disease."

> *No matter what she has forgotten, Anna still lights up when she sees her two grandchildren. I always tell my five year old that Grandma can no longer use her memory like we do, but her heart still works just fine. — Alissa*

> *We explained her illness to the grandkids as an "owie" in her head that sometimes makes her say and do silly things. — Leslie*

Grandchildren who see their grandparent frequently (or, perhaps, live with their grandparent) will be witnessing the disease (and the changes) on a regular basis. Depending on their age, you may need to explain the disease in greater depth, and talk with them as the disease, and their grandparent, changes. Grandchildren who live at a distance, or rarely see their grandparent, may only need a general overview of the disease and updates on an as-needed basis.

Caregivers recommend that you:

❑ Assure the grandchild that, unlike a cold, Alzheimer's is not contagious. They can't "catch" it.

❑ Reassure them the disease is no one's fault. Children sometimes feel responsible for things that happen within a family.

❑ Tell them their grandparent has an illness that will cause them to forget things and, in time, act differently. Tell them, as the disease progresses, their grandparent may forget their name and who they are. Assure and re-assure them that if that happens, their grandparent still loves them — and always will — but that the disease makes it difficult for them to remember, or say, the words.

❑ Remind the grandchild that *you* love them — and always will.

❑ Explain that Alzheimer's is a long, drawn-out illness and that, over time, things will change and people may get exhausted, confused and short-tempered but you will always do your very best to love and care for their grandparent — and them.

❑ Be honest and tell them you don't have all the answers. Tell them even the doctors and experts don't have all the answers about Alzheimer's.

❑ Encourage and allow them to talk to you and express their feelings. Acknowledge their feelings and don't ever judge or criticize what they are saying or how they feel.

❑ Continue to provide opportunities, and time, for them to talk, ask questions or express their feelings about their grandparent and Alzheimer's.

❑ Tell them whatever they are feeling is absolutely normal.

❑ Watch for changes in the grandchild's behavior since they can be indicators as to how they are handling everything. They may begin to act out or withdraw — either at home, at school or with their friends. They may become irritable, impatient or sleep more or they may begin to complain of headaches or stomachaches. These changes can indicate they are having difficulty processing what is happening or dealing with their feelings and emotions. Talk with them. Find a support group or, if need be, a professional they can talk to.

❑ If your child has difficulty discussing their feelings, you may want to find a few age-appropriate books for them to read and then talk about what they learned from the book or how the book made them feel.

Teach the grandchild to be patient. Tell them they may need to remind their grandparent who they are and where they live — and that they may need to do this every time they visit and several times during the visit. Warn them their grandparent's filters may disappear and, in the process, their language can drastically change and they may hear or see their grandparent doing something they never thought they would. And finally, tell them to be creative. They may want to bring pictures or photo albums. Or they can draw pictures while they're visiting and leave them so their grandparent has a "visitor" even when no one is there. — Roberta

Teens and Alzheimer's

Talking to teenagers about Alzheimer's can be more complicated since their concerns and questions may be more complex and they may want more in-depth information and specifics about Alzheimer's. Therefore, it's important to be prepared in advance of your conversation with your teenager.

Jeanne Kessler is a registered nurse who has worked in the field of gerontology for over 20 years. While serving as the Director of Volunteer Services for the Alzheimer's Resource Center of Connecticut, she developed the Care Camp program which helps teens learn about Alzheimer's. Based on Jeanne's experience in her Care Camp workshops, here is her advice and perspective on grandchildren, teenagers and Alzheimer's.

In my workshops with teens, I cover basic truths about Alzheimer's disease, including:
- Teens don't — and can't — get the disease because it's a disease that strikes older adults.
- Not every older adult gets Alzheimer's.
- Memory loss is not a normal part of aging.
- Since we are all individuals, the disease affects every person differently.
- Alzheimer's affects a person's brain and, therefore, their thinking, memory and behavior.
- There is no cure for Alzheimer's.

One question that typically comes up with older teens (or those who have a relative with Alzheimer's) is if other family members will get Alzheimer's. They're mainly concerned about a genetic link. I tell them what the experts are saying based on the most recent research and findings. I also encourage them to take an active role in their own physical and mental health and do a session on nutrition, exercise and safety.

An important part of the workshop is taking the teens to a facility where they interact with individuals who have Alzheimer's. For some, it is their first experience with the disease so we have a discussion in advance of our visit. I explain the different stages of the disease and that individuals at the facility may range from the early to moderate stage of Alzheimer's (and possibly a few in the later stages). I also focus on the positives of an individual being in a facility.

I explain that a disease doesn't define a person and that the people we visit are individuals who happen to have Alzheimer's. We discuss how we are all individuals with different likes and dislikes. To get them to really understand the concept of individuality, I have them each make a name tag. On their name tag, they place stickers of things they love — perhaps a soccer ball or a dog.

I have the staff at the Alzheimer's facility do the same with the residents and, at our first get-together, everyone wears their name tag. It gives the teens a visual cue and connection with residents who like the same things. It's also a great conversation starter.

I think most teens think they are going to be uncomfortable around the Alzheimer's patients and are uncertain initially about what to say or do. However, I've found that after providing them with some knowledge about the disease, their interaction is usually very successful. I give them lots of encouragement and feedback and we do fun activities with the residents — dance, movement or a ball toss. Once the teens see the residents smiling and enjoying themselves, they relax.

If we have time, I have the kids interview a resident about their life. I have a family member present to answer questions or fill in any gaps so the kids can write a "life story" or put together a collage about the person. It is an extremely meaningful activity because it really helps the teens see who the person was before Alzheimer's — and who they still are, in spite of the disease.

The more a grandchild is taught about Alzheimer's and encouraged to be involved in their grandparent's care, the better they do. I always have a few teens in my workshop who have a grandparent with Alzheimer's, and the feedback I get from them is that they not only learned a lot but are also much more comfortable around — and with — their grandparent. Many say when their grandparent gets angry or mad they now understand it wasn't because of anything they did and also know what to do for them.

Oftentimes, the kids end up educating their parents about the disease or how to handle different situations or behaviors. It's been my experience that kids see the glass as "half full" and, if given the right information and explanation, are less fearful than most adults around individuals with Alzheimer's.

Jeanne Kessler, RN, BSN, is the founder and owner of Care Camp for Kids.

Spending Time With Their Grandparent

Some grandchildren say as soon as their grandparent was diagnosed they began spending more time with them. Others withdrew, saying they were extremely uncomfortable around their grandparent and some eventually stopped visiting their grandparent altogether.

If you see a grandchild beginning to appear uncomfortable or avoiding visits with their grandparent, talk with him or her. Perhaps what they need isn't less time with their grandparent but more understanding about the disease and their grandparent. By talking with them, you'll be able to figure out what the real issues are and how to handle them.

The simple act of spending time with their grandparent may be healing and comforting to a grandchild. And sometimes a grandchild can reach a grandparent in a way no one else can.

Kurtis and his grandfather had a special bond. I'm not sure how or why it developed but it was very noticeable to everyone. Kurtis seemed to have just the right "touch" with

*his grandfather and, as the disease progressed, he under-
stood what his grandfather needed. My father was always a
very proud man and wanted to do everything himself yet,
when he became unsteady on his feet, he'd hold Kurtis's
arm. It was priceless to see an eleven-year-old child taking
his grandfather's hand and guiding him through a restaurant or escorting him to the restroom. He let Kurtis order
meals for him in restaurants which none of us — including
his wife — was allowed to do.* — **Shirley**

Some grandchildren found it helpful to have a special project to
work on with their grandparent, such as:

- One grandson went through family pictures with his grandfather and, if there were people he didn't know or recognize, he asked his grandfather and wrote their names down
so that, in the years to come, the family would know who
the people were.

- One granddaughter went through her grandmother's house
and asked her about all of the antiques and special items.
She put notes on everything so the family would always
know why each item was special to her grandmother.

- Another granddaughter said her grandmother was a great
cook but had never written any of her recipes down. She
spent time cooking with her grandmother and, one-by-one,
wrote down all of her grandmother's recipes. She then had
the recipes made into a cookbook that she gave to everyone
in the family.

- Several grandchildren created a memory book with their
grandparent. It included old photos and memorabilia along
with letters and pictures from family and friends. In addition to being a wonderful project together, the book helped
their grandparent recall events from the past.

- A few grandchildren used a video cameras to interview
their grandparent or made a video with (or about) them.

- Many grandchildren created a special ritual with their
grandparent. For example, every Wednesday they would go
for a walk or play cards together.

A GRANDCHILD'S JOURNEY:
In Their Own Words

In the following section, in their own words, grandchildren will share their story and journey with their grandparent and Alzheimer's.

CAROLE'S JOURNEY: Glad I Took The Time

When my grandfather was 88 years old, he fell from a ladder while pruning a tree. After he was released from the hospital, he went to live with my aunt. Along with a full-time nurse, she took care of my grandfather and I helped however I could.

Since my great-grandmother had exhibited many of the same behaviors, our family was somewhat prepared. However, my grandfather's descent into Alzheimer's was very quick.

My aunt did the best she could but eventually it became too difficult for her to continue to care for him at home so my grandfather was moved into a nursing home. He constantly walked the halls looking for his car or a bus so he could get out of there. That was really difficult for me — that and when he no longer recognized us.

My grandfather was almost 92 when he died. Toward the end, I made sure I went to the nursing home several times a week to visit and feed him. Even though he didn't know who I was, I'm glad I took the time to visit him, be with him and make sure he was cared for.

My advice to other grandchildren is to keep in touch with your grandparent. Some people find it difficult to watch their grandparent deteriorate. Others think, since the person no longer knows you or realizes you're there, that there's no reason to visit. Push all of that aside and be there. Just be there for — and with — them.

CASSIE'S JOURNEY: I Wish I'd Known More

The first few years after my grandmother was diagnosed with Alzheimer's, my grandfather was her only caregiver. Even though

I loved my grandmother, I didn't want to visit her because of my grandfather. He didn't understand the disease or my grandmother's behavior and was very short-tempered with her. It felt abusive to me and I didn't want to be around that. Eventually, I began to visit my grandmother, but only when she was alone or if my grandfather was at work (he worked a few days a week at a funeral home).

Alzheimer's completely changed my grandmother. She said and did things she never had before and watching her go through this transformation was very difficult. I remember once, when I was alone with her, she got very angry and told me I was trying to be like "them," the ones "controlling her" (meaning my mother and grandfather). I went into the other room and cried. She soon forgot about it but I never did. It was the first time she'd ever been angry with me and I'd never felt so much anger from my grandmother.

Once, my grandparents gave me money to buy some new clothes for school. When I got home, I modeled the clothes for them. My grandma told me over and over how nice I looked but every time she said it she called me by the wrong name. I finally asked her, "Grandma, what's my name?" but she got it wrong again. Over time, it got worse until, eventually, she forgot who everyone was. At one point, she even thought my grandfather was her father.

In the final years of my grandmother's life, my mother was her primary caregiver. I was working and going to school but I visited her several times a week. She loved when we watched movies together. She always loved to paint so I bought some color-by-number paint sets but she had too much trouble understanding what to do.

You could tell my grandmother knew something was wrong because she would apologize for how she was and sometimes she'd cry about it. Sometimes I'd catch her staring off into space but if I asked what she was staring at, she wouldn't respond. I'd say her name to get her attention but she would just look away. She never responded. Other times I'd ask my grandmother what she was thinking about and she'd say, "About you." That always melted my heart. She always told me how beautiful I was and how proud she was of me.

I remember the last day I looked into her eyes. It was a Monday afternoon. I told her I loved her, and she (barely) mouthed "I love you, too" back to me. Those are the last words I ever heard her say, and the last time I made eye contact with her. I will never forget that moment. A week later she slipped into a deep sleep and never woke up.

Handling the loss of my grandmother has been both easy, and difficult, for me. I know my grandmother isn't in pain and is finally free of her bodily prison, but I miss her dearly. I think about her all the time. I dream about her and, in my dreams, she is always young and healthy.

I'm grateful my family kept my grandmother at home during her illness. I do wish I'd known more about Alzheimer's, especially the advanced stages, so I could have been better prepared. I also wish I'd cried more with my mom because we both needed it.

My advice to other grandchildren would be:

- Spend time with your grandparent. Your time with them is really much shorter than you think. I really appreciate the moments I had with my grandmother.

- You may learn more about your grandparent than you ever thought possible. I found out more about my grandmother through this experience than I had known about her in all the years before Alzheimer's.

- It's hard work, but you won't regret — or forget — this experience.

- Prepare and educate yourself. Learn about the disease or there's a chance that different things will scare you. Know, too, that it's normal to be scared, shocked, sad or angry. Don't hold it in.

- Friends may try to be there for you but they won't always understand.

- Your grandparent may say or do things you never thought they would. They may also forget your name or who you are. Remember, it's the disease.

- Consider participating in the Alzheimer's Association's Memory Walk. I had no idea, until I walked for the first time, how many people are affected by Alzheimer's.

- Most importantly, tell your grandparent you love them.

DEBRA'S JOURNEY: Both My Grandmothers Had Alzheimer's

Both of my grandmothers were diagnosed with Alzheimer's very near the end of their lives. I'm an occupational therapist so I knew as soon as my grandmothers began repeating things and getting confused it was because of Alzheimer's.

My main concerns were for my grandmothers' safety and for my grandfathers. I helped and supported them any way I could but taking care of my grandmothers definitely took its toll on both of my grandfathers. They were both completely dedicated to caring for their wives and they persevered through some very difficult times.

After my grandmothers died, my relationship with both of my grandfathers grew stronger. We called or wrote and spent as much time together as possible. One of my grandfathers bought a little red pickup truck and, since he'd been unable to go anywhere while my grandmother was alive, he and I (and my newborn son) travelled around in his truck visiting people he hadn't seen in years. We also spent a lot of time looking through pictures and he told me a lot about their life together and what my grandmother was like as a young woman.

I was lucky to have had such a long relationship with all of my grandparents. They all lived very long, full lives. They always took care of me so anything I did at the end of their lives wasn't a chore, but an opportunity to watch over them like they had always watched over me.

If I were going to offer any advice to others grandchildren, it would be:

- Don't think there's anything you can (or will) do that will ever undo the effects of Alzheimer's.

- Remember your grandparent isn't being stubborn or defiant. It's the disease.
- Be kind.
- Take care of yourself — and remind your parent (or any other caregiver) to do the same.
- Make sure, as much as possible, that your grandparent is eating healthy food and getting exercise.
- Enjoy your grandparent and enjoy your relationship. Even though things have changed, you are still a family. Be a family and remember the role of every family member isn't to cure your grandparent, but to love them.

♡

HEATHER'S JOURNEY: Both My Grandfather and Father Have Alzheimer's

My grandfather, Jichan (Japanese for "grandfather"), was diagnosed with Alzheimer's when I was 15. Since my grandmother had died many years before, my mother became my grandfather's caregiver.

I lived at home for the first few years and helped out with day-to-day tasks. In the beginning, my grandfather was still fairly self-sufficient and insisted on going home to do his woodwork and gardening. It was great to see him staying so active. However, we didn't want to leave him home alone at night so I drove him back and forth every day. Eventually, he moved in with us.

I was in college at the time and, even though my mother kept me updated by phone, it was hard when I came home from college to see the changes in him. They weren't always drastic changes but even watching the little things slip away hurt.

Every morning, we gave my grandfather the newspaper with his breakfast and he would flip through the pages. We all thought he was no longer able to read but one day we asked my grandfather to read a birthday card — and he did. I think that was one of the happiest moments I had in a long time — knowing my grandfather still had the ability to read — even if just a few words.

My father has now been diagnosed with Alzheimer's, too. My mother is now caring for two people she loves who both have

Alzheimer's and it has completely changed her life. Unless someone can stay with them, or help her, Mom doesn't leave the house. Everything my mother does revolves around my grandfather and my dad. She doesn't do anything for herself anymore.

My mom is doing what is right for both her father and husband yet she still does everything in her power to keep my sister and me as a top priority in her life. I don't know how she does it. I think she's amazing.

If I were going to offer any advice to other grandchildren, it would be:

- Remember that Alzheimer's is different for every person so you really can't predict what path the disease will take. Also know that your grandparent might become a completely different person.

- Don't underestimate your grandparent. Just because they've slowed down, or aren't as sharp as they used to be, they're still capable of doing things that will surprise you.

- Encourage your grandparent to do things for themselves for as long as possible — simple things like buttoning their own shirt or brushing their teeth. It will take longer but allowing them to do it will enable them to hold onto that skill a little while longer.

- Look through family photo albums with your grandparent. Play backgammon or memory games. Do anything they enjoy that will help keep them alert and thinking.

- Even when it's hard, smile — and try to get them to smile.

- There's nothing easy about this disease. It's hard work — and more so emotionally than physically. As much as you may want to — or think — you can do it by yourself, you need people to help you.

JENNIE'S JOURNEY: My Concerns Constantly Changed

I was 17 when my grandmother, my mother's mother, was diagnosed with Alzheimer's. Shortly after her diagnosis, my grandmother moved in with us and my mother became her primary caregiver.

I was a senior in high school and, as much as it pains me to say this, my initial concerns were primarily for myself. I was a teenager who was used to getting all of my parents' attention and I wasn't prepared to have an "older sister" who would take up so much of my parents' (especially my mother's) time and attention. It was a difficult adjustment for me.

After I went away to college, my concern shifted to my parents since they were caring for my grandmother while also running a business full-time from our home.

My grandmother lived with us for four and a half years but, as the Alzheimer's progressed, it became increasingly difficult to keep her safe. My mother finally decided to move her into an assisted living facility one mile from our house.

My concern then shifted to my grandmother. I can't imagine how difficult it must have been for her to no longer be living with us. Even though my mother visited my grandmother every day, I worried because I knew the quality of care wasn't always the best — and certainly not what my mother had been providing for her.

A few days before my grandmother was transferred to hospice, I was sitting holding her hands and talking with her. She looked at me and said, "I love you, Jennie." I couldn't remember the last time she'd said my name. After all of the hard times, and the roller coaster ride we were on at the end of her life, this single moment made the entire journey worth it. It will be a memory of my grandmother I will always cherish.

Looking back, I wish I hadn't been so afraid, angry, or annoyed over having to spend time with my grandmother. It was difficult to communicate with her and, since I found the whole situation rather frightening, I avoided it (and my grandmother) as much as possible. At the time it seemed like the best option. I also wish I'd been more patient.

$\heartsuit$

KAREN'S JOURNEY: Still Grandma

I was honored to be able to care for my grandmother since, after my mother's sudden death, she and I had become a "team." I quit my job to take care of my grandmother and, initially, I thought she would get better with proper and sufficient care. However, in small increments, my grandmother got more and more confused until she became completely helpless and had to be strapped into a wheelchair.

She was 89, unable to speak and incontinent. She had lost all interest in watching her television programs or doing cross-stitch or crossword puzzles. I struggled with the grief of losing Grandma as I had known her before and I also felt completely alone.

One afternoon, when I was feeling particularly down, I started to cry and told my Grandma what I was feeling. I didn't expect her to understand or respond since she seemed totally caught up in the past and had begun calling me by my mother's name. Therefore, it surprised me when she said, in a very present and resolved voice, "Well, I guess I need to be like I was back then."

Astonished, I looked into her eyes and caught a glimmer of the woman she'd been all of her life. Here she was, in the midst of disabilities and hallucinations, trying to comfort me and be the person I wanted her to be. From then on, I began to find the small ways she was still the Grandma I had always known.

To other grandchildren: you will learn things about yourself and life. Despite Alzheimer's, my grandmother still taught me valuable lessons.

KRISTINA'S JOURNEY: Alzheimer's Destroyed The Family We Had

My grandmother was diagnosed with Alzheimer's shortly after my grandfather died. My grandfather had been the center of my grandmother's life and, after he passed, we began to notice she was becoming more forgetful. She would lose her train of thought or get lost in the town where they had raised all three of their children.

Nanny (as I called her) was 79 when she was diagnosed. I was 25 and a mom. It was our family's first experience with the disease.

Initially, my Aunt Rosanne was her primary caregiver and cared for Nanny at home with the help of a nurse's aide. I helped care for Nanny and her house and, since she always loved children, I took her several times a week to my son's school or sporting activities.

It was a difficult time because there was constant bickering in the family over the level and quality of care Nanny was receiving. Family members disagreed over what steps needed to be taken next or argued over who was going to be responsible for taking care of my grandmother, her house or her savings. Alzheimer's, and what my grandmother was going through, destroyed the family we had before her diagnosis.

After Nanny had surgery for a bleeding intestine, she was completely bedridden and in the midst of full-blown Alzheimer's. Some believe the anesthesia worsened the Alzheimer's but, regardless, a decision was made to move her to a nursing home.

Even with others now responsible for Nanny's care, things within our family didn't improve. Family members still weren't getting along so, at the request of the nursing home, we had a family meeting. The meeting didn't go as smoothly as it could have and, from that point forward, the facility tried to work individually with family members to honor our wishes while also making the best decisions for my grandmother.

I was concerned for my grandmother. I was worried she wasn't receiving the same level of care we had provided for her at home or that she might be hurt or harmed while in the facility. My aunt and I went to the nursing home every morning to visit and bathe my grandmother and, many days, I stopped by after work, too.

Most mornings, my aunt and I spent our time just having fun with Nanny. We curled her hair and put beautiful pink lipstick on her lips. We surrounded her with pictures of things she loved and we laughed together. It was the only way we knew to get through it all.

I never knew what to expect when I walked in. Some days Nanny was more "with it" than others. Those were days of happiness and hope — days that reminded me who my grandmother was before Alzheimer's. But there were other days, too — days filled with rage, anger, misery and pain. There were days when my grandmother was constantly looking for her deceased mother and sister. Even though my aunt, my cousin and I were the people she was closest to, she yearned for the family she had grown up with and who had already passed.

Nanny loved my son but, towards the end, I limited his visits with her. She no longer knew his name or that he was her great grandson. She only knew him as a beautiful child. I could feel his pain and that, combined with my own pain, was too much to bear.

Nanny was the matriarch of our family and after an entire life spent working as a nurse and caring for others, she went from being my vibrant, nurturing, old fashioned Catholic-Italian grandmother who had devoted her life to her friends, patients and family to a child who needed constant attention and care. I'm forever grateful my Aunt Rosanne, my cousin Heather and I were all physically able to make the most of every minute of Nanny's life and to be there for her when she needed our strength and love the most. Our focus was on enjoying our time with her and comforting her to the end

Alzheimer's slowly breaks everyone's heart. It was such a difficult couple of years that I lost sight of how much I would miss Nanny when she was gone. At the same time, I'm happy I spent as much time with her as I did when she needed me the most.

To other grandchildren, I offer the following bits of advice:

- Find humor in answering questions multiple times.
- Be sympathetic and respectful of your grandparent. Remember, they're struggling too.
- Surround your grandparent with things they love, even if it's just pictures. It helps for them to have something to focus on.
- Remind them who you are as much as you need to — and never forget who they are to you.
- Tell them constantly that you love them even if they don't say it back.
- Always talk to them like they are the person you remember. You may be shocked when one day they reply or say something that surprises you or makes you laugh.
- Keep them involved with your life and your family.

♡

MAX'S JOURNEY: Our Lives Revolved Around Caring for Great Grams

I was eight years old when my great-grandmother was diagnosed with Alzheimer's. It was my first experience with the disease.

Great Grams, as we called her, was 89. She was my mother's grandmother and a widow.

My family always knew we would take care of Great Grams since she had made it very clear she never wanted to be in a nursing facility. She moved into our house and my mom and dad, my grandmother and grandfather and I all took care of her. I don't have any brothers or sisters.

Everything in our lives revolved around caring for Great Grams. We accepted that she was one of us and included her in everything and took her everywhere, but taking care of her during the last two years of her life was very difficult.

I wish I'd known that extreme paranoia is fairly common with Alzheimer's because I got very upset when Great Grams had delusions. She tried to run away because she believed we were going to kill her. She told strangers, hotel guests, police officers, and repairmen who came to our house that her life was in danger because we were trying to kill her.

Eight months before she died, we all went to Hawaii. On the trip, Great Grams ran off and told a security guard we were trying to kill her. We ended up meeting a lot of native Hawaiians on that trip, namely the Honolulu police department. It hurt because I knew how hard we were all working to take care of Great Grams but I also understood it was part of the disease.

My parents were also worried about my grandmother. Since Great Grams wasn't sleeping, and wandered around at night, both my grandmother and great-grandmother weren't getting any sleep. Sometimes, my grandfather slept on the floor in front of Great Grams' bedroom so my grandmother could get a few hours sleep.

The doctors began to tell us Great Grams should no longer be cared for at home and insisted she needed skilled care in a nursing facility. They also said her memory medication was no longer helping her and as soon as they took Great Grams off her medication, her decline was immediate and massive. If we had it to do over, we would have kept her on the medication.

Even after Great Grams went into the nursing facility, we still planned on bringing her home to care for her but it was not to be. She died within a few months and just before her 93rd birthday.

I think we all did the best we could in caring for Great Grams and I'm happy we kept her home with us as long as we did.

Alzheimer's, and my Great Grams, made a huge difference in my life. I now have a goal of becoming a geriatric psychiatrist so I can spend my life helping others. And I also founded a non-profit, Puzzles To Remember, and am helping many people with Alzheimer's disease and dementia across the country.

I would tell other grandchildren that taking care of someone with Alzheimer's is very difficult but also very rewarding. You will come out of the experience a more mature, empathetic and stronger person.

MIKE'S JOURNEY: Alzheimer's Is A Terrible Disease

Alzheimer's is a terrible disease. People who have a family member with cancer (or other disease) have hope. With other diseases, it can often be treated, the person can be cured, and the disease may never come back. That can't and won't happen with Alzheimer's.

With Alzheimer's, it's like watching one of your family members wither away mentally, and then physically, into nothing. The strongest part of my grandmother — her mind — was being taken from her and there was absolutely nothing I or anyone could do to stop it.

I was a teenager when my grandmother was diagnosed and my mother helped my grandfather care for her. Even though my mother was with my grandparents a lot, I can't say I ever felt abandoned or neglected. It didn't bother me that my mom wasn't home all of the time because I understood, and still understand, what she had to do and I absolutely respect her for it. If anything, it made me feel better when I saw her dedication to both of her parents.

I have a tendency to avoid spending time with people I think (or know) are dying. It's a self-defense mechanism and makes it easier for me to cope with the eventual loss of someone I love. However, looking back, I wish I'd spent more time with my grandmother.

The other thing I would have done differently is tell my mother and grandfather more often what an amazing job they did caring for my grandmother. I can't believe, watching all they went through, that they were able to keep their sanity. Honestly, the hardest part of Alzheimer's for me was not only watching what my grandmother was going through but also watching the toll it took on both my grandfather and my mother.

I will always remember Thanksgiving 2007. We knew my grandmother was dying so my mother, my brother and I were in her room talking to her. My grandfather walked in and I remember he looked at my grandmother and smiled. It was obvious the smile was a cover for what he was really feeling because I could see the sadness in his eyes. I will never forget that image. It haunts me to this day to know what this disease can do — not just to those who have the disease but to those who love them the most.

My advice to other grandchildren is to spend time with your grandparent. Also support the caregivers and remind them to take care of themselves.

SEAN'S JOURNEY: What Happened Was A Tragedy

When it started out — when Grandmom was first diagnosed — it wasn't so bad. She would forget a word or forget she'd just told you a story and repeat it. It was actually kinda cute. But then it got worse and there's nothing funny or cute about your grand-mother not remembering her family or how to eat.

Honestly, what happened to my grandparents was a tragedy. My grandmother lost her memories, her motor skills and, eventu-ally, her life. And my grandfather lost the woman who he described as "his life." They say that bad things happen to good people and what happened to my grandparents is a perfect example.

To other grandchildren, I would offer the following bits of advice:

- Roll with the punches. If your grandparent tells you the same story a million times, smile and listen.

- When my grandmother forgot her own name, I would smile and say, "Hey, lady." It was a simple word she still remembered and could relate to.

- Likewise, if your grandparent forgets who you are — or your name — don't make a big deal of it. Tell your grandparent your name or let them call you something simple and generic. Having my grandmother smile and call me "her boy" was still comforting, even during the final stages of her illness.

- Try to stay positive and focus on supporting family members who may be caring for your grandparent.

Three Siblings, Two Grandmothers and a Journey with Alzheimer's

Kelly, Bryan and Devon are siblings. Both of their grandmothers were diagnosed with Alzheimer's but, because of the difference in their ages and where they were at in their personal lives, their experience with their grandmothers and the disease was quite different. We'll begin by hearing from the oldest of the three, Kelly.

Kelly:

I was a teenager when Grandma R. (my mom's mother) was diagnosed with Alzheimer's. Several years later, when I was in my early 20s, Grandma K. (my father's mother) was diagnosed with the disease. Both of my grandmothers lived in New Jersey but I was living in Seattle, 3000 miles away, so I only got to see them once a year when I visited for a week.

It was difficult coming home and not knowing how to be with a grandparent you rarely saw who was now in a totally different state of mind. I just went along with whatever mood they were in and understood it was the disease, not them, and I continued to love them.

On one trip home, I took Grandma R. for a chemo treatment.

She had breast cancer and her doctor told me the Alzheimer's was helping her get through her treatments miraculously well. Since she was basically clueless that she was sick with either disease, it helped her stay stress-free and happy through what could have been a very stressful time. That was a powerful example to me of the mind-body connection.

I have two memories of Grandma K. that always put a smile on my face. One is her dancing a polka to the "Chicken Dance" song. The other is when she looked at my boyfriend, Bill (who has since become my husband) and told me she could see in his eyes how much he loved me. I feel as though the disease brought out a wonderful simplicity in her. She took the time to be playful and silly and appreciated love wherever she saw it.

As the disease progressed, I was concerned my grandmothers would become "someone else" and that everyone would forget the loving women they were their entire lives.

I was also concerned that my parents weren't taking care of themselves. I knew how painful it was for them to watch the sad transformation of their once-strong parent. I also knew it put a strain on both of my grandfathers. I was sorry I wasn't closer to help. Even though I talked with everyone by phone as much as possible, I would have liked to been able to hug them more regularly.

Both families are big-hearted and loving. I believe caring for my grandmothers was a natural extension of who they are and what they would do for any member of their family. I respect them for stepping up and supporting all of my grandparents and am grateful to be a part of two amazing families.

If I were going to offer advice to someone who has a grandparent with Alzheimer's, it would be to:

- Be there for both your grandparents and parents.
- Expect a full range of physical, emotional and spiritual demands on your family.
- Realize that your grandparent will always be the same person inside but, eventually, the disease will make them unrecognizable. Try to remember the core of who they are/were.
- Take time to process your own feelings.

Bryan is three years younger than Kelly. After graduating from Virginia Tech, he moved to Seattle, near Kelly. Both of his grandmothers, by that point, were well into the disease. Here's what Bryan says about those years.

Bryan:

I loved both of my grandmothers very much and it was hard to see them, basically, lose their minds. My only regret, in retrospect, was my lack of involvement through the tough times at the end of their lives. I was either away at school or living across the country but, when I was around, I tried to do as much as I could to provide support to lighten everyone's load and lift their spirits.

While I tried to remain positive and help as much as I could, I also removed myself from the situation especially as my grandmothers' health and memory declined. A lot of that had to do with being frightened or uncomfortable with seeing my grandmothers in such a helpless state. It was hard to see two strong-minded women, who were such a huge part of my life when I was growing up, to now be at the total mercy of such a debilitating disease.

Both of my parents' lives were fairly consumed by caring for their mothers. I could see how much it affected and aged them in just a few short years. It was tough to see the frustration and pain they went through. I wanted to help but didn't have a clue what I could do. It was a tremendously hard sacrifice they made. I hope, if someday I'm faced with a similar situation, I'll be able to rise to the challenge like they did. I was proud of all they did and the sacrifices they made. I just wish it all could have been avoided somehow.

I'd encourage other grandchildren to:

- Spend as much time as you can with your grandparent.
- Enjoy time together while you still have it.
- Make the process as easy as possible for your grandparent, your parent and yourself.

♡

Devon is the youngest of the three siblings. She was 14 when her Grandma R. was diagnosed with Alzheimer's. It was her first experience with Alzheimer's. Devon was the one, out of all three siblings, who was the most involved with her grandmother's care.

Devon:

My grandmother was in her mid-70s when she was diagnosed with Alzheimer's. She was an orphan at a very young age so there was no way to know what, if any, illness or disease (such as Alzheimer's) she may have been genetically predisposed to.

While I wasn't involved with any of the caregiving decisions, I overheard the discussions. There was a lot of turmoil and opposing feelings about what was the best way to care for my grandmother. In the end, even though everyone understood the hardships involved in having my grandfather care for her, they also understood it would have been more painful for him to have her taken out of the home and cared for by someone else. So my grandmother remained at home and my grandfather took care of her. His three daughters — my mom and two of her sisters — helped as did another granddaughter and I.

I was very involved in my grandmother's day-to-day personal care, including:

- **Showering** — I wanted my grandmother to maintain some sort of independence for as long as she could so when it was time for her to take a shower, I stood outside the shower, leaving the door mostly ajar. I handed her the soap and showed her (in mime) where and how to lather and rinse. If I saw that she was getting frustrated, I took over. I could tell when she reached that point because she would look at me with childlike eyes that said, "How do I wash myself?" The role reversal was quite astounding for me because I'm sure I gave her the same look when I was young and unsure how to do something.
- **Toileting** — including cleaning up after accidents.

- **Feeding** — Towards the end, mealtime became a tedious and stressful process because my grandmother was paranoid and believed her food had been poisoned. Since I knew fear can be a part of Alzheimer's, I spoke to her in a sweet, lulling voice to calm her down. It usually worked and sometimes I was the only person who could get her to eat. Towards the very end, despite all of our best efforts, even getting my grandmother to drink required extraordinary patience.

- **Blood/Sugar Tests** — since my grandmother was also a diabetic.

- **Medication** — I helped administer my grandmother's oral medications. After she passed, we found a muffin pan in the oven filled with her pills. Apparently, my grandmother held her pills in her mouth and then, when we weren't looking, took them out of her mouth and into the muffin pan.

- **Moral Support and Love** — I kept kindness, love and respect in my heart and let that guide my demeanor and actions with all of my grandparents.

Sometimes my grandmother would get upset and say, "You know, I'm in here somewhere," pointing to her head. I never felt so hollow in my life. It reminded me of the scene in the movie *The Exorcist,* when they lift up the little girl's shirt to see the words "Help Me" being scribbled across her belly from the inside out. To think that my grandmother was aware of her situation and was somehow trapped inside herself was horrifying.

Caring for my grandmother was hard at times so I had to allow myself to enjoy the more light-hearted, amusing and heart-warming moments. A perfect example was during a period when my grandmother was resisting food, she still woke up in the middle of the night to eat cookies. Despite all she no longer remembered, she never forgot where the cookie jar was. You had to laugh.

There were also beautiful experiences with my grandmother brought on by Alzheimer's. When I hugged my grandmother, she would lay her head on my shoulder, coo and linger in my embrace.

We were a very affectionate family but, before Alzheimer's, I never held my grandmother like that. I think her decline into complete dependency caused an almost childlike affection. Those moments are so precious to me now.

At the same time, I worried about my grandfather. It was hard to see this illness overtaking my grandmother and, in some ways, my grandfather, too. It was such an extraordinary struggle for him and he got increasingly depressed and often felt helpless and frustrated. It was as if he was clinging to my grandmother's body even though she very seldom resembled the person he had been in love with for so many years. Despite the pain it caused him to see her that way, I believe my grandfather would have held onto my grandmother's body forever if he could have just to see her face or hear her voice. When you have spent a lifetime with one person, it must be hard to separate their life and sufferings from your own. I really thought my grandfather wasn't going to be able to go on without my grandmother. Even though he has, I think a huge piece of him died with her.

I was young and even though it was scary and painful, I was never fearful for myself. Because of Alzheimer's, I shared a profound experience with my grandmother and she had grown even dearer to my heart. I thought I was mentally prepared for her death because, obviously, we all saw it coming but, in the end, I wasn't prepared at all. To this day, I still struggle with her death.

This experience impacted my life on so many levels. It gave me a more defining notion of family. After witnessing the daily outpouring of love my grandfather, mom, and aunts bestowed on my grandmother, I realize there is nothing more beautiful than a family functioning as a unit, carrying and caring for each other, as they carry — and care for — one of their own.

I don't believe I will ever have anything to be more proud of in my life — or do anything as important — as taking care of my grandmother. HANDS DOWN. NO COMPETITION. PERIOD. I feel blessed to have been a part of it.

If I were to offer any advice or insight to other grandchildren, it would be:

- The experience will make you more aware of your own personal strengths.
- Cherish the small, miniscule moments with the people you love.
- It helps to remember to laugh.

Chapter

7

Joy In Your Journey

It may be difficult to comprehend how, or why, someone could use the word *joy* or *gratitude* in the same sentence as the word *Alzheimer's*. Yet amidst the chaos, confusion and angst of Alzheimer's, there are also moments of extreme tenderness, compassion and love. Those moments sustain caregivers and are the sacred moments they treasure.

Caregivers say finding joy in their journey usually came about through a deliberate shift in their thinking about Alzheimer's, their parent, and themselves.

FINDING JOY IN YOUR JOURNEY

1. Begin With an Attitude of Gratitude

2. Accept and Embrace Change

3. Laugh!

4. Live In — and Cherish — The Moment

JOY-FULL STEP #1: Begin with an Attitude of Gratitude

Caring for your parent can mean days filled with endless concerns and moments of anxiety or exhaustion. How, in the midst of all that, do you find the time, energy or inspiration to be grateful?

Caregivers say it begins by intentionally choosing to focus on the things you are grateful for in your life. Many say it helps to physically and mentally stop at least once a day to review your day — and to think about the things for which you are grateful. To help you do that, many caregivers suggest using one simple tool: a Gratitude Journal.

A Gratitude Journal

A Gratitude Journal is a journal where you write down things for which you are grateful. It doesn't matter if your Gratitude Journal is a simple pad of paper or a beautiful blank journal. It only matters that it's convenient to use and something you'll enjoy writing in.

It also doesn't matter where or when you write, but it *does* matter that you write on a regular basis — and preferably every day.

Some caregivers keep their Gratitude Journal with them and write in it throughout the day. Others keep it on their nightstand and write in it every morning when they wake up or at night before going to bed. Some caregivers write three things, some write one, others keep going until they can't think of anything else to write.

One caregiver wrote on small pieces of paper that she posted around her house — on her bathroom mirror, the refrigerator, or next to the coffee pot. By seeing and reading the notes while she brushed her teeth or made a cup of coffee, it allowed her to begin her day remembering the blessings and special moments that had already occurred. It also got her mind focused on gratitude.

Some caregivers combined regular journaling (like we discussed in Chapter Four) with their Gratitude Journal. They began with regular journaling — writing down anything they wanted and anything that was on their mind. By writing about any pent-up frustrations or emotions, it was easier to then transition to writing things for which they were grateful. They also said, by ending on a positive note, it allowed them to start (or end) their day focused on the blessings, rather than the demands, of caring for their parent.

Initially, many caregivers say they struggled with writing in their Gratitude Journal but, over time, it got easier. They say by knowing they had to find *something* to write, it kept them aware of — and looking for — individual moments and blessings throughout their day. That awareness helped them realize that even the most difficult days have moments of lightness and joy.

As you keep writing, your thinking and awareness will shift and so, too, will your attitude and approach to your parent. You may find yourself looking for creating and holding onto the simple, heart-filled moments with your parent. By becoming more aware of these moments, you may gain a new understanding and appreciation of your parent, Alzheimer's and caregiving. It may also allow you to remember what you still have with your parent, rather than on what you are losing (or have already lost) because of Alzheimer's.

Studies show that regularly expressing gratitude and focusing on the positive can:

- Change your perspective.
- Restore a sense of optimism, energy and enthusiasm.
- Provide a greater sense of well-being.

Try keeping a Gratitude Journal for one month — 30 days — and see what happens.

I learned to focus on the successes, rather than the stresses, of the day. Every night before I laid my head on the pillow, I found one "victory" to be thankful for and one thing which made me laugh. Sometimes it may have been a small victory like having only one pill spit out at me instead of all of them. By finding something every day to celebrate, instead of focusing on the daily disasters or emotional overload, it kept my spirits up and helped me maintain my sanity. Looking for something that made me laugh helped me notice the funny side of Alzheimer's. Like the day Mom, who was 88 at the time, just knew she was in labor and having a baby when it was actually me who was eight months pregnant. — **Chris**

♡

I am grateful every time I enter my mother's room and she still knows me and I see the love in her eyes. — **Donna**

♡

Before Mom was diagnosed with Alzheimer's, I led women's workshops. One of the things I had the women do was keep a Gratitude Journal. It's something I learned from the Oprah Winfrey Show. It had been helpful for me and every single woman in my workshop found it to be helpful in shifting her thinking and focus.

After Mom was diagnosed, I continued to write in my Gratitude Journal. But, after a while, I put the journal in my drawer since it was becoming increasingly difficult for me to write in it. Most days I was on the verge of exhaustion and the Gratitude Journal felt like one more thing to do in a day that was already filled to overflowing.

Then one day I ran into a woman who had taken my workshop. She told me how much her life had changed since we met at my workshop and how helpful it had been for her to write in her Gratitude Journal.

That night, I took my Gratitude Journal out of the drawer and started writing in it again. The first few days I struggled to find anything to write. In fact, more than once, I wrote "I'm grateful I made it through the day and I'm still in one piece." But I remembered the importance of sticking with it and every day it got easier. Once again, my thinking shifted. I found myself looking for, and being more aware of, the good (rather than the bad) moments throughout the day. It changed the way I approached the day and my mother.

Now that Mom is gone, I'm grateful I kept my Gratitude Journal. It's amazing how, simply by reading an entry, I'm taken back to a special time or place with her — a smile or a joke we shared or an afternoon sitting on her deck watching the squirrels together. It helps me remember the good times — and there were a lot of good times. — Patti

JOY-FULL STEP #2:
Accept — and Embrace — Change

Life with Alzheimer's can mean subtle and sometimes not so subtle changes. Since no one can stop the changes from occurring, what caregivers *can* do is accept and embrace the changes, and the "new" life and person (parent) standing before you.

Many caregivers shared stories of how the changes brought about by Alzheimer's allowed them to see a new side of, or gain new insights into, their parent. Some heard details of stories never before shared in their family. For some, the changes brought about by Alzheimer's allow them to know and embrace their parent on a deeper, and more meaningful, level.

My father-in-law, Dan, died in May 2004. My mother-in-law, Anna, was with him when he died but she was a very private person and never spoke of his death.

Anna came to live with us in 2008. One day, Anna began to tell me in vivid detail about the moments leading up to, and the moment of, Dan's death. She told me she was sitting next to his hospital bed, holding his hand, when Dan asked her if he was dying. She said she told him he was and that it was okay to go toward the light and be with his parents and siblings who had already passed.

"Tommy will take care of me," she assured Dan. "It's alright for you to go."

And, with that, Anna said, Dan closed his eyes, took his last breath and died. She told me he had a smile on his face and looked so peaceful. Anna had never been one to show much emotion. Yet, when she was recounting those moments, her voice quivered and she was overcome with emotion.

*We never again spoke of the day Dan died and today Anna has no recollection of her husband. However, I'm grateful for that brief moment when she told me about those final moments with Dan. To be honest, I don't know if I would have ever heard about it if it hadn't been for Alzheimer's. — **Alissa***

Since Mom was always very embarrassed by her overbite, she rarely smiled with her mouth open. However, after Alzheimer's, she became almost childlike and, on several occasions, laughed and smiled freely and without embarrassment.

*We also gained some of our biggest insights about Mom as a result of Alzheimer's. As Mom relived the earlier years of her life, we learned a lot about her and those years through her "young eyes." It was really wonderful to see how happy she'd been during that period of her life. — **Ann***

I had never wanted to be in the same room as my mother-in-law because she was always so bitter but, through her journey with Alzheimer's, I watched her change and become a nicer person. Even though she no longer recognized me, or anybody else in her life, she smiled at us. Gone was the harsh look on her face. Gone was the sarcasm, the bitterness, the venom, the chiseled look of years of self-induced misery, hatred, and holding grudges. She forgot the reasons why she hated people; she forgot about her difficult childhood, the rejection she'd experienced, and the people who hurt her. Instead, she experienced each day anew. She said "please" and "thank you." She smiled. She sang. She laughed. She said "I love you," and she meant it. It was pure and from her heart. There were no ulterior motives. Alzheimer's brought peace and comfort to a truly wounded soul.

Closely guarded secrets she'd held inside for so long

innocently came out because of Alzheimer's. I learned she'd been molested as a child and had an intense fear of abandonment. I realized there were reasons for her bitterness and that it was simply a defense mechanism. She was simply trying to protect herself from ever being hurt again.

As my mother-in-law changed, so did I. I learned to love her and also developed a compassion for her which I'd never had before. I finally understood that her difficult childhood had clouded her adult life. I finally understood the hostility in her, and what that hostility had done to my husband during his childhood. Through the things I've been shown on this journey, I found joy and understanding and, through that understanding, I learned to forgive. I also finally found peace in my relationship with my husband. — **Chris**

♡

Before Alzheimer's, my father wasn't one to hug or show affection either at home or in public. When my mother hugged him, he would chuckle and pull back, embarrassed by the attention. Whenever I hugged or kissed him on the cheek, he would sit, very stiff, and tolerate it. However, after Dad progressed into the moderate stage of Alzheimer's, he got quieter and didn't talk as much — but he also now enjoyed getting a hug or kiss and having his hand held.

One Sunday, we were all at my brother's house when my mother decided it was time to leave. She said her goodbyes and moved towards the door. Dad lagged behind so we all took turns saying goodbye and hugging and kissing him. Mom finally said, "Robert, it's time to go. Stop stalling and come on."

Without hesitation, my father said, "I think I'll stay here. I like getting hugs." — **Shirley**

JOY-FULL STEP #3: Laugh!

In 1981, former *Saturday Review* editor Norman Cousins wrote a book titled *Anatomy of an Illness*. In it, Cousins describes being diagnosed with ankylosing spondylitis — a degenerative, crippling and irreversible spinal condition. By following non-traditional methods, including reading humorous books and watching comedies — including classic Marx Brothers films — Cousins was able to reduce his pain level and ultimately triumphed over his illness. His book, and story, were one of the first real-life examples of using one's mind as a tool for healing and using humor to boost the body's capacity to heal.

Since then other studies and individuals have revealed, time after time, that King Solomon was right when he said "a cheerful heart is good medicine."

> *"My belief is that we are going to eventually discover that the most dramatic health benefits of humor are not in laughter, but in the cognitive and emotional management that humorous experiences provide. The experience relieves emotional distress and assists in changing negative thinking patterns."* **— Steven M. Sultanoff, PhD, Clinical Psychologist**

Neuroscientists have documented that laughing, humor and play can stimulate the immune system, lower stress hormones, relax muscles, ease anxiety and fear, improve mood, strengthen relationships and diffuse conflict.

One may think a diagnosis of Alzheimer's means there is no longer anything to laugh about. However, as a social worker and specialist in therapeutic laughter, I have found that laughter and maintaining a sense of humor not only helps the families cope but helps the patients thrive as well.

Laughter, just like crying or other forms of expressing emotion, is a valuable coping tool. It helps release the tension often associated with fear, anger or grief and clears the way for the caregiver to maintain a connection with their parent.

During my work at an in-patient behavioral unit, I was asked to conduct weekly laughter sessions for Alzheimer's and dementia patients. In addition to relaxation breathing and stretching, we laughed. We didn't tell jokes or try to make people laugh. We simply laughed for no reason. Often patients, who no longer spoke or made eye contact, would begin to smile or clap.

I remember one gentleman who refused to engage in any activities. Instead, he sat, sulking, in his chair. At the first session, he was unwilling to participate. I didn't force him but I did try to encourage him. That afternoon, like every afternoon, he began pacing. However, the staff was amazed when he began clapping and saying, "Ha! Ha! Ha!" — the exact words we'd used in that morning's laughter session. As the staff laughed and smiled with him, the tension was eased and a connection was made.

When your parent laughs, smile and laugh with them. When they tell a story, find the humor in it and giggle. Embrace laughter and enjoy the moment.

Lynn Shaw, MSW, LCSW, specializes in laughter therapy for stress resiliency. She is also an Assistant Professor in Human Services at Ivy Tech Community College in Indianapolis, Indiana.

Alzheimer's changed Dad's personality. He used to be very quiet and anxious but is now very witty and laughs a lot more. He's given my husband and me many good laughs and I've actually kept a log filled with the funny, cute and special comments Dad's made. Here are a few of the entries from the "funny log":

- *Dad and I were riding in the car one day when we began talking about dogs. I told him I loved dogs but we were too busy and didn't have the time to dedicate to a dog right now. "Yes, they need a lot of attention," he said, then smiled and added, "And I do, too!"*

- *Gratefully, Dad has a good appetite and, most nights, enjoys his dinner. After dinner, he'll smile and say, "Okay, I think I'll stay another day!"*

- *Today's weather report was "hazy, hot and humid" with a heat advisory. The weatherman suggested people check on the elderly and small children. Dad just laughed and said, "You better check on me!"*

- *I forgot to pick something up from the store today and, when I told Dad, he laughed and said, "Uh-oh. Looks like I have to get someone better." I think it makes him feel a little less frustrated about his own memory issues when he knows I have trouble with mine. — Allyson*

After Mom went to a facility, she would show up in someone else's clothes or I would see Mom's clothing on other people. You can't get upset over things like that. We learned to see the humor in it and would often make a game of trying to see how many people would have Mom's clothes on in any given day. — Dorothy

I remember once when the phone rang and Mom answered the TV remote control that was lying on the coffee table. She not only answered it but proceeded to have a conversation with it! Know that it's okay to laugh and also important to find the humor in everyday situations. — Jaye

We have a lovely large Victorian home which has been our family's "holiday center" since my children were little. I am fortunate that my grown children have always been able to come home for Christmas. It became especially important when we realized my mom, their only surviving Grandma, would soon be gone from us.

Mom had recently moved to a nursing home but we were still able to take her out for special occasions. My dad wanted to make the holiday nice for Mom and took extra care in getting her ready for the holiday. He made sure Mom had her hair done earlier in the week and brought her a nice outfit from home. He shopped so Mom would have gifts to give everyone. We were all excited to have a chance to give Mom some joy and to experience it together while she was still somewhat able to understand.

Mom hadn't eaten meat or had a drop of wine for decades. But at dinner that year, she gleefully stole a piece of turkey from my Dad's plate laughing at us when we gasped. We were delighted to give her all the turkey she wanted and after she emptied her goblet of sparkling fruit juice, she held her glass up for a refill. She kept moving her glass and laughing when we went to fill it. She finally laughed and said, "I want what Jesus made — wine!" We were astounded, but gladly complied. Even though she wanted more, we kept it to one glass.

When it came time to open presents, we all gathered around the tree. We have always been rather civilized about our gift opening. We designate a "Santa" who gives each person one gift. When everyone has a present, one by one we open our gift for all to see and thank the giver. When round one is complete, the process starts again until all presents have been opened.

This Christmas, Mom wasn't about to wait. She was like a mischievous child when the first present was handed to her. She eagerly ripped into it, completely disregarding our ritual. We all laughed. After her first present was open, she handed it to my Dad and looked for the next one. We started giving her presents to open just so we could watch her giggle and laugh. The present was irrelevant to her, it was the opening she enjoyed, so we let her open as many as she wanted. Mom was such a serious and somber person and this persona was totally new to us.

We hadn't known what to expect that year. The fun and laughter became a precious gift and memory for all of us to enjoy as Mom began to withdraw more and more. Eventually, it became too stressful for her to leave the nursing home, so on her final Christmas, we played Santa at the nursing home. After we left, my daughter cried and said she didn't want to do that any-

more. She wanted to remember the "Christmas of Laughter" with Grandma. — Jayme

⤙ ⑤ ⤚

JOY-FULL STEP #4:
Live in — and Cherish — The Moment

Alzheimer's brings with it a world of uncertainty and unpredictability so, for caregivers, it's easy to worry about what tomorrow holds. If your parent forgets a close friend's name one day, you may wonder if they'll forget your name the next day. However, by fretting and worrying about yesterday or tomorrow you may miss the simple joy of today.

Mary M., a caregiver for her mother, said the secret is to: *"Live in the moment...and cherish each one"* and the following stories from caregivers are beautiful examples of doing just that.

I vividly remember one particular visit with Mom. When I arrived, Mom was telling an aide how much she loved her. A gentleman approached them with his therapy dog and Mom began fawning over the dog. She was having a wonderful time. In recent weeks, Mom had become anxious, talking about Daddy and constantly wanting to go to Alabama. But today, there was no hint of any of that.

As I approached Mom, she looked at me and immediately said she was ready to go back to her room to begin "packing for Alabama." My heart sank.

In her room, I saw two pictures stacked on her nightstand and her blanket and wrap folded on the end of the bed. She was ready to go, she said, and would be leaving in the morning.

Since Mom doesn't think about leaving when she's out-of-sight of her belongings, I steered her back out of her room and down the hall to the dayroom. There, a woman sat at the table with a jigsaw puzzle. Not a single piece had been put into place.

She asked Mom if she'd help her put the puzzle together and, since Mom loves puzzles, she jumped at the chance. Every time Mom fit two pieces together, the woman congratulated her and Mom got excited. For the moment, Mom forgot all about Alabama.

When Mom finished the puzzle, she said she was ready to "go to the house." We walked back to her room where she again started talking about going to Alabama. I began telling her stories and jokes and, for a few moments, Mom was distracted.

In the end, all any of us has is this moment. After my mother was diagnosed, I decided that every day she knew who I was would be a good day. So far, they have all been good days. I know in time that will change but, until then, I'm grateful for the moment. — Alan

♡

My mother-in-law, Anna, lived with us for half of my daughter Ella's life and the two of them became best friends. They would hold hands at the store or sit together for hours looking at photo albums. Whenever Ella was mad at my husband or me, she would tattle on us to Grandma. I always loved hearing Ella, Anna and my son, Adam laughing when they played together. Anna no longer remembers but my children still talk about "farming on the floor" with Grandma.

I feel blessed that my kids had one of their grandparents live with them and, despite all Anna has forgotten, she still lights up when she sees Adam and Ella.

What became important for us was to stop trying to create new memories (which Anna wouldn't remember). Instead, we focused on making great moments for her and our efforts were compensated by seeing a big smile on her face or seeing her completely enthralled by something. We understood and accepted she wouldn't remember it in a few hours (or, possibly, a few minutes). But in that moment, Anna was having a great time. It was the moments that mattered for her and for us. — Alissa

♡

Some of my most precious memories revolve around my grandmother and ice cream. Growing up, we didn't always have ice cream at my house so my grandmother always kept ice cream in her freezer for me. It was a special treat we shared.

One day, after my grandmother was bedridden and unable to do anything for herself, I made a big bowl of vanilla ice cream and strawberries and sat and shared it with my grandmother. I still remember the smile on her face. To this day, anytime I have ice cream, I'm instantly reminded of the comfort of my grandmother. — **Cassie**

I loved the little moments. I loved taking my father-in-law to lunch with his sisters-in-law and watching the four of them together. I loved taking him dancing. I thought it was cute that he never realized he was washing the same plastic dishes over and over. I loved how he made me laugh when he tried to pay for a meal with the fake money I gave him. I just loved taking care of him. — **Marie**

Dad is just so pleasant. When we go out for lunch, he's always eating "the best burger" and if we're out for a drive or a walk, the trees are always "the most beautiful trees."

One day, we were outside and there was a bush teeming with bees. There were bees everywhere but on one branch sat a butterfly. As we got closer to the bush, my mother said, "Oh, look at all the bees."

My father smiled and said, "And look at the butterfly."

Alzheimer's has changed my Dad. He's more relaxed and happier. He notices things he never did — and things the rest of us sometimes miss. He sees things, and life, differently now. He's a joy to be with. — **Sue**

This story is about my uncle who had Alzheimer's. It still makes me cry to think about this.

Aunt Alma and Uncle Bob were involved in a major car accident. My uncle only ended up with a broken toe but my aunt suffered brain damage, along with other physical problems, and was unconscious for a long time. After recovering from his injury, my uncle retired and took care of my aunt in their home. A real act of love!

Over the years, my cousins noticed my uncle was becoming more and more forgetful. Initially, they thought it was just the pressure of taking care of my aunt but ultimately it was determined that he had Alzheimer's.

Gratefully, he didn't understand the diagnosis meant he would no longer be his wife's primary caregiver since he believed caring for her was part of the vows he had taken when they were married.

A caregiver was brought in for both my aunt and uncle but as the Alzheimer's progressed, my uncle became a "wanderer." He would walk out the door and they'd have to go find him. Eventually, it became too unsafe for my uncle to continue living at home, so he was put into a nursing home.

The last time I saw Uncle Bob was at an anniversary party they had for him and Aunt Alma. At that point, he'd been in the nursing home for about a year and, since my aunt was unable to get around very well, they hadn't seen very much of one another.

When Uncle Bob arrived at the party, I was surprised he no longer knew anyone — his grandchildren, his children — nobody except Aunt Alma.

Uncle Bob walked straight up to Aunt Alma, called her "Sweetie" and asked if she was okay and if she had a boyfriend. Aunt Alma was the only one Uncle Bob knew the entire day.

That moment had an enormous impact on me and made a huge difference in my life. It made me understand, on a whole new level, that no matter what happens, love prevails. —Jerry

Chapter

8

Looking Back On Their Journey

I asked our caregivers to look back on their journey and answer the following questions:

1. What do you wish someone had told you about Alzheimer's?
2. What do you think you (and/or your family) did right?
3. What would you have done differently?
4. What would you want other sons and daughters to know about loving and caring for a parent with Alzheimer's?
5. How have you been changed by your experience with your parent and Alzheimer's?

Here is what they said.

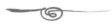

QUESTION #1: *What do you wish someone had told you about Alzheimer's?*

I wish someone had told me:

- not to argue with an Alzheimer's patient.
- how to cope with raising two small children while caring for someone who no longer knew who her son was, let alone me or the children. — *Alissa*

I wish someone had told me:

- to take the time and find a support group that's a good fit.

- not to listen to everyone. There are things I wish I had done, but didn't, because I was basing my decision on someone else's experience.

- just because somebody recommends something doesn't mean it's a good idea. When I was moving Mom into an assisted living facility, a "professional" told me, "Pretend you're taking her to lunch." It was the worst advice I ever received.

- to never move anyone you love into a facility on a Friday because weekends are understaffed. — *Ami*

I wish someone had told me:

- allowing your parent to think they are in the past with a loved one isn't a bad thing.

- your parent can have a "game face" they use to mask the disease or symptoms of the disease. — *Ann*

I wish someone had told me:

- to really look at the terms of your long-term care insurance. Our long term-care insurance only really helped if the increase in monthly costs was contained and if the care was provided for a certain period of time and in a variety of living situations.

- how difficult it is to lose someone piece by piece.

- you'll have days when you'll actually be jealous of friends who have lost their parents. — *Chanah*

I wish someone had told me:

- that getting along with staff at every level of daycare, in-home care, the nursing home, hospitals, and rehab requires patience, confidence in your decision-making, a building of trust on both sides, and a watchful eye over every person and process.

- how incredibly difficult it would be to try and be an interesting companion to my father on a daily basis when I hadn't lived with him for 25 years.

- the most valuable thing I could do was separate my father from the disease.
- how to handle my father's physical needs (e.g., getting in a car, sitting in a chair, eating). — *Charlie*

I wish someone had been able to give me a glimpse of life in my mother's shoes. — *Chris*

I wish someone had told me Mama would know there was something wrong. — *Grace*

I wish someone had told me:

- this disease is not just about your parent, but the whole family. It can thoroughly break a family.
- caring for your parent and the caregiver's *emotional* well-being is just as important as meeting their *physical* needs.
- responding appropriately to your parent's outbursts and anger is critical. — *Janice*

I wish someone had told me:

- it's not like the movie *The Notebook*.
- you may lose the chance to make amends, ask necessary questions, express gratitude or forgiveness, or say goodbye before you even realized you wanted or needed to.
- you could come to a point where you don't want to see or visit your parent because it feels like they're already gone.
- you might be afraid you'll end up just like your parent — confused with a loss of dignity, waiting and wanting to die, and having no control over any aspect of your life. — *Jayme*

I wish someone had told me:

- living with Alzheimer's is a very, very expensive condition for which there is little (or no) medical insurance reimbursement.
- I was about to embark on the longest and most life-changing journey of my life.
- there are worse things than dying. — *Kitty*

I wish someone had told me:

- how bad the mood swings can be and that my once calm and loving mother could become shockingly mean.
- to seek support immediately. I bottled things up and tried doing everything myself. It was until it was all over that I realized how much of a toll it had on me.
- that my mother could be very crafty and cover up the illness. — *Leslie*

I wish someone had told me:

- how much strength you need to get through this.
- the importance of learning as much as you can about the disease.
- how frustrating it is to deal with hospitals and nursing homes who only see your parent as another old person. — *Pat*

I wish someone had told me:

- the physical, mental, psychological and spiritual toll Alzheimer's has on the caregiver.
- ways to better support my dad while he was caring for my mother.
- how much it would hurt when my mother no longer knew who I or my sons were. — *Patti*

I wish someone had told me:

- to give Dad the same gentle love and attention I would give a child.
- to not take it personally if your parent yells or doesn't recognize you.
- to be patient and breathe. — *Sabrina*

I wish someone had told me:

- simple medical issues (like a urinary tract infection) can cause dramatic and sudden negative behaviors.
- Alzheimer's eventually results in an inability to drink liquids.
- most family doctors and general practitioners don't know

anything about Alzheimer's and won't necessarily refer you to people who do.

- music can reach patients who have lost the ability to use their voice in conversation. — *Shirley*

I wish someone had told me:

- sometimes the "experts" aren't experts at all and that medical professionals don't necessarily understand Alzheimer's or how to treat Alzheimer's patients.
- the transition between stages isn't always a gentle progression but can be like falling off a cliff.
- this is a very expensive disease, especially if you're no longer able to care for your parent. — **Victoria**

I wish someone had told me to find the humor in things. — **Wanda**

QUESTION #2: *What do you think you (and/or your family) did right?*

- We found a good doctor who specialized in Alzheimer's.
- We e-mailed the doctor before every visit so she knew what was going on.
- We involved Mom in everything our family did.
- We arranged for art classes and created a tap dance class.
- We trained a service dog for Mom.
- We traveled for as long as Mom was able.
- After moving Mom 60 miles away from her social circle, we installed an 800 number so her friends could call her toll-free.
- We made sure Mom felt she was contributing to the family.
- We made sure she had a "job" to do (sewing quilts, dye painting fabric).
- I reminded myself Mom wasn't doing this to push my buttons.
- We lived in her reality and didn't argue.

- I understood Mom needed to feel able and capable more than I needed to obsess about what other people might think of her. — *Ami*

We went along with her fantasies that my brother and father were alive. We lived in the moment with her. We laughed and tried to keep things light — and we loved Mom unconditionally. — *Ann*

- Our lives — and time — stood still so we could take care of Mom.

- We contacted the appropriate resources and got the information we needed so we knew what we were up against.

- We visited with Mom no matter how tired, exhausted or depressed we were.

- We loved Mom unconditionally...and we cried. — *Barbara N.*

While she still remembered people, places and stories, we went through my mother's pictures and I made a memory book for her. In the process, I got to learn things about my family I never would have known otherwise. — *Chanah*

We learned to focus on the successes rather than the stresses of the day. — *Chris*

We made decisions together as a family. — *Grace*

We listened to my dad's frustrations, pain and anger. It's okay to not have answers. Sometimes people just want to be heard. —*Janice*

We communicated — even though we learned the hard way. We allowed our father to have control of Mom's care until he was physically unable to do so. We believe it helped our father keep his sanity long after life had turned upside down. We also obtained Power of Attorney(s) for both of my parents while they were both still lucid and reasonable. —*Jayme*

I show him every day that I love him. —*Jeannot*

- We got Mom into a program that kept her mentally and socially stimulated which, I believe, helped more than any medication.

- We lined up an assisted living facility before Mom needed it. When the time came, we were ready.
- We kept Mom's routine the same as much as possible.
- We gave her little chores (e.g., folding laundry, cutting coupons, peeling potatoes, etc.) so she felt like she was contributing and part of the family.
- We kept our sense of humor.
- We loved her and told her so all the time. — *Karen B.*

We understood our responsibilities — as well as our own physical and emotional limitations. We were honest with our loved ones who had Alzheimer's — and ourselves — about their condition and prognosis. We became strong, active and vocal advocates for change in both state and federal public policies on issues affecting families and persons with Alzheimer's. — *Kitty*

We kept her involved in family activities and gatherings, even after she moved into the facility, and surrounded her with things she loved — music, animals, children and television. — *Kristina*

- We paid attention to the signs and sought help as soon as possible.
- We admitted she needed to live in a facility to ensure her continued safety and, after she moved into the facility, we monitored everything and visited or called as often as possible.
- We tried to take it one day at a time.
- We told her every chance we got how much we loved her. — *Leslie*

We cared for Dad as a family and kept him home with us. We loved him unconditionally and laughed with him. — **Lois**

We kept Dad at home and socially active for as long as we could. We had family gatherings on a regular basis to try and keep him aware of all of us. — *Pat*

I think we did everything right. I wouldn't change how we did anything. We did the best we could. All of us. — *Sabrina*

We shared and discussed the diagnosis with Dad. — *Shirley*

- We got the legal stuff in order and had a thorough medical workup done as soon as Mom was diagnosed.
- The entire family weighed in on major decisions but we had one person at a time responsible for Mom.
- Mom never spent one day in a hospital or skilled nursing facility that I wasn't there with her. — *Victoria*

We had a plan to take care of everyone, not just Dad. We exploited resources and we celebrated together. — ***Wanda***

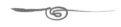

QUESTION #3: *Looking back, what would you have done differently?*

I would have:

- sought counseling to better cope with caring for an Alzheimer's patient.
- attended caregiver support group meetings much sooner.
- explored other options of keeping Mom at home longer. — *Alissa*

I would have:

- moved Mom to a different assisted living facility instead of trying to micro-manage the shortcomings of the one she was in.
- found better live-in help rather than giving up.
- trusted my own instincts instead of listening to the "experts."
- taken better care of myself. I still haven't gone back to the level I was before all this and she's been gone over a year and a half.
- talked to Mom about how she was feeling and what she was thinking rather than assuming I knew best.
- given more of myself to our daughter. I ran out of energy for her.
- I would have tried harder not to feel guilty. — *Ami*

I would have:

- tried to avoid having anyone tell or remind Mom of any troubles in the family or the world.

- done more to encourage Mom for as long as possible. She loved being helpful.

- Also, my daughter said she would have spent more time with her; and my husband said he would have spent less time correcting or arguing with her (even if he knew he was right). — *Ann*

I would have:

- noticed things Mom was doing earlier so we could have caught it sooner.

- not admitted Mom to the hospital while we were waiting for availability at the facility.

- visited Mom more often.

- not been such a nasty teenager to her. — *Barbara N.*

I would have been more involved with Mom's care in the beginning rather than letting my sister do it all. — *Bonnie*

I would have:

- tried to make sure family members were more sensitive to each other.

- taken a more active role in my mother's life.

- explored more options for my mother's care. — *Chanah*

I would have trusted my instincts earlier — and bit my tongue even more than I did. — *Gayle*

I would have sought help earlier and done more research on what was available through the Veterans Administration. —*Jeannot*

I would have:

- been more assertive with my father-in-law in order to help him understand the care he was providing to my mother-in-law was only depleting his financial resources and prolonging her (and his) suffering.

- asked (and allowed) my daughters for their help and assistance with my husband earlier and more often.
- done oral histories with both my mother-in-law and husband and been more proactive in taking the time to capture memories while they were somewhat intact.
- celebrated each coherent day with them a little more.
- kept a personal journal. — *Kitty*

I would have:

- admitted her illness to friends and family sooner; and realized that, by telling them, I wasn't embarrassing or dishonoring Mom.
- tried to see things from her perspective and understand how terrified she must have been in the early stages.
- most importantly, I would have shown her more patience, especially in the beginning. — *Leslie*

I would have:

- researched nursing homes far in advance of Dad needing one.
- known more about programs and help available to families of veterans.
- kept someone in Dad's hospital room at all times.
- insisted that no drugs be given to Dad without having full prior knowledge of their side effects. — *Pat*

I would have:

- done more with my dad before the disease advanced.
- asked my dad what he wanted after he was diagnosed.
- let go of the tears sooner. — *Rhonda*

I would have:

- transitioned Mother from living in her home of 18 years directly to the Alzheimer's assisted living facility without the intermediate stop in assisted living.
- fought harder to get the hospice diagnosis sooner.
- taken Mother to another hospital so her care could be handled by a different medical group. — *Victoria*

QUESTION #4: What would you want other sons and daughters to know about loving and caring for a parent with Alzheimer's?

I'd want others to know:

- redirecting your parent's attention to something else when they are agitated works really well.

- Alzheimer's patients have no idea what yesterday was or what tomorrow may bring. They live fully in the moment. It's up to you to create moments for them to enjoy — knowing once the moment is gone, so is their memory of it.

- your parent is still a human being and deserves respect and dignity. — *Alissa*

I'd want others to know:

- to pace yourself. Alzheimer's is a marathon, not a sprint.

- you need to be a strong advocate for your parent. Don't let other people push you or your parent around. — *Ami*

I'd want others to know that even if your parent can't speak or say your name, they can still sense your presence and know your face. — *Barbara N.*

I'd want others to know:

- you need patience — lots and lots of patience!

- even if you and your parent have a bad day together, hug and kiss them goodnight.

- they are still your parent, even if you're now the one caring for them.

- you need to laugh more and cry less because there's nothing you can do to stop what's happening to them. Laughter is healthy.

- you need to keep things in perspective. Life is too short to worry about small things. — *Bonnie*

I'd want other to know:

- ignorance is not bliss. Denial of the illness may keep you from taking advantage of resources available to you and your parent.
- Alzheimer's is likely to push family issues onto the front burner. Be aware of, and sensitive to, the dynamics within your family.
- your parent may try to cover up their memory loss and lack of judgment. The more social skills they have, the more likely they are to do it and the better they will be at it.
- if your parent starts calling everyone "dear" (or another generic name), it may be a warning sign.
- there is a fine line between giving your parent autonomy and not allowing them to get into situations that could be potentially harmful or dangerous.
- you should learn how to communicate with your parent.
- you need to take care of yourself. There is a reason why many caregivers predecease the person they are taking care of. Get support! — *Chanah*

I'd want others to know:

- you need to find a mutual respect and build trust with any professional caregivers you work with.
- while your parent's behavior may appear childlike, they are still adults and deserve to be treated as such. Don't treat your parent like a child.
- you don't have to be afraid to laugh and tell jokes and have a good time. Your parent may not understand the joke but they will still pick up on the positive energy, laughter and smiles.
- you need to put yourself in your parent's shoes. If you're out for a walk, does your parent need sunglasses, a hat or sunblock? If you're pushing them in a wheelchair, ask if they're cold or would like a sweater or blanket. Remind your parent to drink water (or give them something to drink) on a regular basis. They may be thirsty but not

know how to ask for it — or even know they need or want it. In other words, constantly put yourself in your parent's shoes and ask yourself "What would I want in this situation?" — *Charlie*

I'd want others to know:

- your children are learning an important life lesson about honoring and loving a parent, in good times and bad, by watching you care for your parent.
- there is an end to the disease. The journey can be excruciatingly slow at times but it will end. — *Chris*

I'd want others to know it's important to be sure your parent is in a safe environment and to constantly reevaluate if there needs to be a change in their living arrangement (especially if they're living alone). — *Dorothy and Kathy*

I'd want others to know there are things like aromatherapy and Bach Rescue Remedy that can help relieve your parent's symptoms and behaviors, and also help keep you calm. My sister regularly used a lavender spray in the house and put drops of Rescue Remedy in Dad's water — or rubbed the cream into his hands while giving him a hand massage. It helped keep everyone calmer, especially when Dad went through a particularly difficult phase. — *Frank*

I'd want others to know:

- it's important to love and appreciate every moment you have with your parent.
- it's very tough and sometimes frustrating — and you can come away feeling angry and somewhat robbed.
- the whole "parenting your parent" can seem very odd at first but eventually can become very natural. — *Janice*

I'd want others to know:

- it helps to be patient, stay positive and keep your sense of humor.
- to listen with your ears, see with your eyes but understand with your heart.

- a hug goes a long way. — *Jaye*

I'd want others to know that it's important to practice compassion and patience. — *Jayme*

I'd want others to know:

- sometimes it's not that others don't *want* to help but that they don't know *how* to help or what to do.
- you shouldn't be afraid of, or feel guilty about, placing your parent in care settings other than your home. Know that whatever decision you make is harder on you than it is on your parent.
- you shouldn't be ashamed or embarrassed about Alzheimer's. — *Kitty*

I'd want others to know the importance of nurturing yourself every day. Take care of yourself — emotionally, spiritually and physically. — *Laura*

I'd want others to know it's important to be optimistic but also realistic. — *Pat*

I'd want others to know:

- this disease can break your heart one second and, two seconds later, mend it with a special moment shared with your parent.
- it helps to think about things from your parent's reality. Think how scary and confusing the world must be for them.
- you're going to grieve a little bit every day as your parent slips away and then, in the end, you'll grieve all over again.
- it's important to focus on things you can still do with your parent. You can still laugh with your mother, go for a walk with your father, or share a hug or special moment with them.
- on your toughest days, love will carry you; and, in the end, love is all that matters. — *Patti*

I'd want others to know the importance of having all the legal documents prepared after your parent is first diagnosed. Things were so much easier because my parents signed all the necessary papers early on, including Do Not Resuscitate (DNR) orders and Power of Attorney (POA) for both health and personal property. Since I was named POA, when my mother (who was my father's caregiver) broke her ankle and was unable to care for him for a long time, I was able to step in and get him the care he needed and also get everything ready for Mom to approve and sign. — *Sabrina*

I'd want others to know:

- There's a natural tendency to get mad or angry at the situation and direct that anger at your parent. Remember your parent can't help what has happened to them.
- You should seek out support groups. You're going to need a shoulder to cry on. — *Sandie*

I'd want others to know:

- it's important to get past denial as quickly as possible, so you and your parent can meet the challenge of Alzheimer's head-on and enlist all the resources available to you.
- you need to arm yourself with knowledge and be proactive for your parent in every aspect of their life.
- Alzheimer's is nothing to be ashamed of.
- things are not always as they seem. Try to really understand what your parent is reacting to by putting yourself in their shoes. — *Shirley*

I'd want others to know:

- not to hold everyone to your standards. Every family member or friend will make their own choices on what they're willing to do and acknowledge and they alone will live with those choices in the future.
- only you can embarrass yourself. There's nothing anyone else can do or say that reflects on you and should cause you embarrassment. — *Susan*

I'd want others to know:

- you don't know what kind of care your parent is getting in a facility unless you're there frequently.

- you can't count on help from Medicaid.
- if your parent is engaging in sexual activity with someone else at a facility you may not have the right to know the other person's HIV status.
- it's important to get on very good terms with the administrator of the facility where your parent lives. If your parent becomes troublesome, they might get the benefit of the doubt. — *Victoria*

I'd want others to know:

- there's something funny in every situation. Try to find it.
- your parent is forgetting the bad along with the good. — *Wanda*

QUESTION #5: How have you been changed by your experience with your parent and Alzheimer's?

I realize I can no longer take memories I hold dear for granted. Before Alzheimer's, I would say, "I'll never forget that for the rest of my life." Now, after living with Alzheimer's and seeing what my mother-in-law went through, I say, "I hope I never forget that."

Because of Alzheimer's, I learned the strength of my relationship with my husband. I truly believe after all he and I have been through with his mom and this disease, we can make it through anything. — *Alissa*

Because of Alzheimer's, my sister and I had a communication breakthrough and are much closer. Alzheimer's also gave me a greater appreciation for the elderly as a whole and allowed me to see that even when they're seriously ill, they like to laugh and have fun. — *Charlie*

After my Dad was diagnosed, I started a blog. It wasn't always easy to put into words what we were going through, but I hoped it would allow others to see what a family goes through when their loved one has Alzheimer's. Most people think the disease only affects their memory. They don't know about all of the behaviors or how it affects every fiber of the caregiver's being.

Through my blog, others have come to understand a little more about Alzheimer's.

Since we've been on this journey with Alzheimer's, every little thing I forget makes me wonder if I'm showing signs of the disease. Do I forget more than other people? I have no idea. But if I walk into a room and forget why I'm there, I wonder. If someone tells me an address, and I can't remember it five minutes later, I wonder. If I forget where I put something, I wonder. So I wonder a lot. I always will. Until there's a test to tell me conclusively, I'll wonder. — *Cheryl*

My experience with Alzheimer's has made me a better person. It forced me to have patience with someone who is confused, doesn't understand, constantly repeats something or is just in need. It made me realize that despite a person's outwards appearance or behavior, there is still a person inside along with sparks of who they were or are. Sometimes you just have to work a little harder and be more observant to see it.

I have developed an even deeper love and admiration for my mother. I am constantly amazed at my mother's courage amidst the changes this disease has thrown at her.

I have grown more as a person since this journey with Alzheimer's in these past four years than I had in the previous 20 years — and all for the better. — *Donna*

Alzheimer's taught me patience and taught me to take things not just one day, but sometimes one minute at a time. I did a lot of self-evaluating during this entire process and ultimately I learned understanding and forgiveness — for others as well as for myself. — *Dorothy*

I've done a lot of growing up since Alzheimer's became a part of our lives. I now have a deeper understanding and respect for the elderly. Having my father diagnosed with Alzheimer's has also allowed me to better understand my mother and her feelings. — *Heather*

My grandmother's diagnosis completely changed my life. I am now in a master's program in gerontology. I don't think I ever would have pursued this career path had it not been for my experience with my grandmother and Alzheimer's. — *Jennie*

How has Alzheimer's changed me? Let me count the ways. I've lived with Alzheimer's off and on for over 20 years, but here are some of the "highlights":

- It provided me with a front-row seat on how far we have come in understanding this disease and an even more disturbing understanding of how much more there is to learn before there is a cure.

- It allowed me to make some remarkable friendships around the country with people whose lives, like mine, have been touched by Alzheimer's.

- It shaped my professional career as an advocate and provided me with constructive and meaningful opportunities to educate legislators and policy-makers about some of the many special challenges confronting Alzheimer's patients and their families.

- It helped me become more patient and understanding.

- It exhausted and inspired me.

- It very nearly bankrupted my family.

- It brought an already close family even closer together.

- It broke my heart...twice.

- It confirmed that public hostility toward insurance companies is not misplaced.

- It instilled in me a real (and normal) fear for the uncertain genetic chain into which my children and grandchildren have been born.

- It left me a widow, and alone, much earlier than I ever expected.

- It reminded me that memories are precious and meant to be shared.

- It helped me appreciate and value everything — every day — on a much deeper level. — *Kitty*

Alzheimer's taught me how to help others and also gave me the opportunity to be at my mother's side when she passed. I realize now what a great honor it was to be able to care for my mom. I participate in the Alzheimer's Association's Memory Walk every year in her memory not only because Alzheimer's affected my life but in the hope that someday there will be a cure so no one else has to ever live with this disease. — *Leslie*

Alzheimer's has made me self-conscious of everything. Every day I live with the fear that it will happen to me. Whenever I can't think of a word, remember a name or forget an appointment, it's always in the back of my mind. If I misplace my car keys or forget a small detail, I wonder if it's a sign that I, too, have this horrible disease. I watch my siblings for little signs, too. I think we all now live with the fear of "what if I'm next."

On the other hand, Alzheimer's taught me that life is not forever and to say and do things today. I hold my family closer and tell them I love them more often. I end each phone call by saying "I love you" because I realize there may not be a next time. — **Pat**

I am much more assertive when it comes to my parents' care now. If I don't like how they are being treated, I'll go all the way to the top, if necessary, to get them the treatment and care they deserve. — *Sabrina*

Chapter
9

The End of the Journey

Even though we know Alzheimer's is a progressive, terminal disease, for caregivers it often feels like a journey without end. Many caregivers say when they were told, or realized, they were reaching the end of their journey with their parent — even though all the signs were there — it still came as a shock.

Even though death is a natural part of life, many people find discussing or dealing with the reality of death to be extremely difficult. Like at the beginning of your journey with Alzheimer's, family members may not want to talk about what is happening with your parent.

This is a difficult, and emotional, time for everyone. Family members may be flooded with emotions. Since everyone handles things in their own way, it's important to remain understanding and compassionate of one another.

As you read through the following pages, don't judge yourself (or anyone else) if you are unable to complete any of the suggested steps. Be gentle with yourself — and others — on this next, and last, leg of your journey with your parent and Alzheimer's.

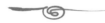

Decisions, Discussions and Documents

There are questions, discussions and documents you and your family might want to consider before you reach the end of your journey with your parent. They are:

- **WHO** will make end-of-life decisions?
- **WHAT** type of end-of-life care will your parent receive?
- **WHEN** will you end treatments?
- **WHERE** do you want your parent to spend their final days?
- **HOW** will you support your parent, yourself, and other family members?

WHO

Ideally, your parent or family has already designated the individual(s) responsible for making end-of-life decisions and has prepared the necessary legal papers to document those decisions.

If not, it's important to consider that some states have laws that clearly identify the chain of command for these decisions if a family hasn't designated otherwise. Typically, the spouse is first, followed by parents, and, finally, children. You may want to check to see what the law is in your state (or the state where your parent resides) or you may want to take the necessary steps to have the documents prepared that would spell out exactly who will be responsible for end-of-life decisions for your parent.

WHAT

The type of care your parent receives at the end of their life can include such things as resuscitation, treatment of other symptoms or illnesses, the use of drugs or surgery, and the use of oxygen, feeding tubes or other life-supporting interventions.

Your parent may have already prepared a medical advance directive, living will or DNR (Do Not Resuscitate) order detailing what type of end-of-life care they want and provided you with copies of those documents. If not, check with your parent's physician or hospital to see if they have any such documents in your parent's medical records.

Make sure all medical, nursing home and hospice personnel

and staff have copies of your parent's medical directives and orders. Make sure they are placed with your parent's charts and records. Keep a copy handy, and accessible, at all times in the event it is needed.

Be forewarned that some medical and other professionals have very strong opinions in this area. These decisions, like so many others, are very personal. There are no "right" or "wrong" decisions. The ultimate goal, as always, is what is the best — and the most loving — for your parent.

Mom's health had begun to deteriorate. She was having problems swallowing and was hospitalized with pneumonia because food had lodged in her lungs.

Her doctor told me it was time to put her on a feeding tube. I told him I wanted both of my siblings to be in on the decision so my brothers and I met with the doctor in Mom's room — and kept in contact with my sister by phone. I had a list of questions to ask the doctor so we could make an informed decision. I really wanted to know details about everything that would happen with whatever choice we made.

We hated seeing Mom bedridden. Was it time to let her go? What quality of life would she have if we put the feeding tube in? What would her death be like if we didn't?

The doctor told us if it was his mother he would put the feeding tube in. He said Mom might build up her strength enough to start walking again and have a better quality of life. We ultimately had the feeding tube put in. As it turned out, the doctor was overly optimistic about what Mom could achieve. She never got any stronger and never walked or talked again.

She did, however, die a very peaceful death with all of her family around her telling family stories and laughing about things that happened in the past. There was so much love in that room when she died. I was holding her hand when she took her last breath and that experience was priceless. My mother brought me into this world and I was grateful that I could be with her when she left it. — Dorothy

WHEN

Along with determining the type of end-of-life care you want for your parent, you also need to consider when you will stop administering life support measures. Again, much of this may already be documented. If not, you and your family need to talk, decide, and have the documents prepared and copies distributed and readily available when — and if — they are needed.

WHERE

Deciding where your parent will spend their last weeks, days and minutes is, again, a very personal decision. Some families want to keep their parent at home so they can ensure they will pass in the privacy and comfort of their own home surrounded by loved ones. Others, unsure how a family member (especially if there are young children in the home) might react to walking in on a loved one who has died, prefer their parent remain in a hospital, nursing home or care facility. Again, there is no right or wrong — only what is right for your parent and your family.

HOW

The final steps on your journey with your parent can be the most demanding, difficult and draining on many levels. In order to care for and support your parent to the end of their journey, it's important that you ask for, and receive, the physical, emotional and spiritual support you, your parent, and your family need from others, including extended family, friends, spiritual/religious leaders or mentors, organizations — or through hospice and palliative care.

WHAT IS HOSPICE & PALLIATIVE CARE?

Hospice provides a holistic approach to a person going through the final stages of their life. Hospice addresses the physical, emotional, psychosocial and spiritual needs of both the patient and their loved ones. Palliative care focuses on pain management and the relief of pain.

Both hospice and palliative care can be provided at a care facility, in a hospital setting or at home. Oftentimes, these services are provided at little or no cost.

*For family members with a loved one at the end stages of Alzheimer's disease, having hospice is a blessing — and as important for the caregiver as it is for the patient. Caregivers may be exhausted from years of providing care to their parent. Many caregivers have socially isolated themselves while providing care and find they have little or no emotional support at a time when they need it the most. Hospice offers support, spiritual guidance and a helping hand on the last part of their caregiving journey. — **Diane Carbo, RN**️*

In my own experience, when our family was told it was time to meet with hospice, I was stunned. At our initial meeting with hospice, I was angry and completely resistant to the idea of having them involved in my mother's care. I knew we didn't need them because Mom wasn't at "that point" yet. I truly believed we still had months, if not years, left with her.

Somewhere along the way, someone had told me that hospice doesn't always mean end of life. They said that some patients actually stabilize under the care of hospice so, even though our hospice nurse and social worker told me that was the exception rather than the rule, I clung to the possibility that it would hold true for us. I clung to every bit of hope and denial left in me.

Our hospice nurse and social worker quietly and gently educated and supported me. As they did, I was finally able to understand, and accept, that Mom's time — and our time with her — was quickly coming to an end.

I'd never witnessed death first-hand and was frightened and unsure of what was happening with my mother but hospice was with me every step of the way. They told me what to look for — the physiological signs that my mother was preparing to leave her earthly body — and what to do. They not only explained what was happening but they showed me how to continue to love and care for my mother in those final days. They also taught me how to let go of my mother with love.

Since I found it both helpful and comforting to know what to look for as my mother approached the end, I am sharing that information with you in the hopes it will ease your burden and help make your final days with your parent easier and more meaningful.

THE SIGNS THAT DEATH IS NEAR

Beginning with the initial onset of Alzheimer's, small parts of your parent begin to die. Over the course of the disease, a series of gradual mini-deaths takes place as you watch your parent's personality change and you watch them lose their ability to speak coherently or remember places and faces. With Alzheimer's, you experience death over and over, day after day, with your parent. Still, no matter how long you have suffered or grieved while watching your parent's decline, when it seems your parent's death is imminent, it can still be a difficult and emotional time.

Caregivers often wonder what signs and symptoms take place in the physical body that point to impending death and what death looks like when it finally comes. The following are natural changes that occur for *all* people as they prepare to die. They may not all be present and may not happen in this particular order; however, they are fairly accurate signs or indicators that death is near.

Decreased Intake of Food and Fluid

As the body prepares itself for death, it begins to slowly relinquish life-sustaining activities, shutting down its functions like a person turning off the lights, room by room, before going to bed.

One of the functions to shut down is the digestive process. Family members often panic when they see that their loved one no longer needs or desires food. Some families want to insert a feeding tube, believing the person they love is starving or dehydrating. But the body is wise. In the dying process, it is taking care to close down functioning in a slow and very deliberate way. There is no discomfort. There is no pain. In fact, if the dying person is forced to eat or drink, it may cause them pain. They can aspirate the food or liquid, causing them to choke or the food may sit in the stomach, undigested, causing discomfort.

The loss of desire — or ability — to eat is a clear sign the person is preparing to leave. When this happens, your family can do several things. First, if your parent is still taking some nourishment, allow them to eat and drink whatever is appetizing to them, but only small bites and sips of liquids should be given. Allow your parent to decide how much or what they want to ingest.

Since your parent's reflexes are slowing down, swallowing may become difficult. Small chips of ice, popsicles or frozen treats may be refreshing to your parent, but again, should not be forced. If your parent has lost their ability to swallow or, if they are no longer taking anything by mouth, swabbing their mouth and lips to keep them moist will help keep them comfortable.

Sleeping

As the body's metabolism slows down, it may be difficult to wake your parent. They may sleep more — and for longer periods of time. It may be comforting for you and your parent if you simply sit and hold their hand, let them know you are there, and talk to them in a quiet, calming tone.

Even if your parent hasn't been responsive in a long time, talk to them. Hearing is the first sense to develop and the last to be lost so tell your parent all the things you'd like them to know. Talk to them as if they were awake. If someone is in the room with you, try not to talk *about* your parent but include your parent in the conversation. You can be assured they will hear you.

Restlessness

As the amount of oxygen in their body decreases, your parent may become restless. They may pull at the sheets or wave their arms. They may grimace, making it look as though they are angry or in pain. This is not the case — it is a normal part of the dying process.

Your parent may speak to you lucidly and tell you they see someone standing by their bed (someone *you* don't see, of course!). Don't be alarmed or interfere or try to restrain them. Talk to them calmly, lightly massage their hand or stroke their forehead or hair, gently. Assure your parent they are fine and that you love them. Playing soft music may also help calm your parent.

Incontinence

Your parent may lose all control of urine and bowels as the muscles in those areas begin to further relax. It's important to keep your parent as clean and comfortable as possible. Your parent's urinary output will decrease and become very dark and similar to the color of tea. Again, don't be alarmed. This is due to the decrease in fluid intake and the lessening of the circulation through the kidneys.

Breathing Changes

Changes in breathing patterns are another indicator that your parent is nearing death. You may notice your parent's breathing becoming shallow, irregular, fast or abnormally slow — with periods of apnea where there is no breathing at all. Your parent may pant or you may hear a moaning sound as they exhale. If this happens, know they are *not* in distress. This is the sound that comes from air passing over their relaxed vocal chords.

Your parent may develop gurgling in his/her chest. This is a normal change and due to a decrease of fluids in the body and inability to cough up normal secretions. It is not causing your parent any discomfort but can be troubling to you or others at their bedside. Since suctioning generally causes more discomfort and often increases the secretions, it's advisable to gently turn your parent's head to the side and allow gravity to drain any buildup of secretions. You should also consider gently wiping your parent's mouth with a moist cloth for comfort.

Color and Pulse Changes

Your parent's arms and legs may become cold, hot or discolored or you may notice their fingertips, toes and lips turn darker with a bluish hue. This is all due to decreased circulation. Since the body is using most of its waning energy for the vital organs, it is no longer circulating blood to the outer extremities.

In addition, your parent's heartbeat and pulse may slow and become weak and irregular. Their temperature may also become irregular and their blood pressure may diminish. These changes indicate the end is very near.

If your parent appears to be cold, warm them with a blanket. Do not use an electric blanket. If your parent is sweating or looks to be uncomfortably hot, cover them with just a light sheet. Keeping your parent as comfortable as possible is all that needs to be done. The body is doing its job exactly as it was created to do. You can support that process by simply being there and calmly and lovingly attending to whatever small needs your parent may have.

Saying Good-Bye

A dying person will sometimes try to hold on, even though it brings them discomfort, in order to be assured those they love will be all right when — and after — they die. Many need permission from the family to go.

It is a blessing for the dying person if their family is able to reassure them they will be fine. It helps the dying person to hear from each family member that they love them, that they will be fine and that they have your permission to leave. A family's ability to reassure and release the dying person is the greatest gift of love they can give at this time. Holding them, stroking them and saying goodbye is also important to those who are left behind. It helps the grieving process tremendously if there is nothing left unsaid.

Death

At the time of death, your parent's breathing and heart will stop and they will be unresponsive. Their eyelids may be partially open and their eyes may be fixed in a stare. Their mouth may fall open as the jaw relaxes. The bowels and bladder may release their contents as the body relaxes.

Crying, talking to, and holding your parent are all perfectly natural and comforting to those who are left behind. This should not be rushed. Sit with the person as long as you need to in order to say your final goodbye. Your parent's body does not have to be moved until you and everyone else in your family are ready.

Depending upon your family's beliefs or culture, you may have a ritual for your parent's death. Some families prepare the body by bathing and dressing it. Others gather around their parent's bedside, join hands and sing or pray. These rituals are healing for those left behind and help them move through grief while also creating a healing connection with the deceased.

Patricia Fares–O'Malley, PhD is a psychologist, educator, international speaker, Bereavement Coordinator for hospice and the author of "Healing The Love Wound."

What Now? Life After Caregiving

For years, your life has been about caring for your parent. It was how you spent your days and dictated many of the choices you made. Chances are you put other pieces of your life on hold — relationships, careers, schooling and perhaps even your health. In many ways, caring for your parent became who you were. Now that your parent has died, who are you? What do you do with your days now that the demands of caregiving no longer exist? What will you do with the rest of your life? How do you go on?

It takes time. Time to accept the finality of your parent's death and time to process the range of emotions you might experience.

Alzheimer's caregivers are sometimes less depressed following the death of their loved one than those who have lost a family member from other causes. Some caregivers also feel a sense of relief. None of this means the caregiver doesn't feel sadness or grief. Rather, it may be a combination of knowing their loved one is finally at peace, the realization that a burden has been lifted, or the fact that they have already been grieving for their parent for years.

Many caregivers have feelings of regret, anger or guilt over things they or their parent could have done differently over the years. They may replay events or moments over in their mind and wonder how it would have been if they had done things differently or if their parent didn't have Alzheimer's.

Try to forgive yourself, your parent, and the disease. Know you did the best you could with the information and knowledge you had at the time. Know that, if everyone had a choice, Alzheimer's wouldn't have been a part of your journey together. Understand that all of these emotions are part of your individual grieving process. Like Alzheimer's, grief is a journey, a process, and can't be rushed. You have to walk through it and know that, one day, you will come out the other side a stronger, wiser person.

*It was difficult caring for Dad, getting him dressed, helping him go to the bathroom, seeing him this way. At the end, I was finally able to get past that and take care of him but, overall, I feel that I let my father down. When the disease got worse, I wasn't there for him when he needed me most. I was not a good son and I will have to live with that for the rest of my life. — **Bill***

♡

Tomorrow will be one year since Dad left this earth. Most people would call me crazy, but there are times I feel his presence. I'll be doing something and, all of a sudden, he pops into my mind for a split second, and it's not the sick person that left this earth, but the Dad I remember.

The next few weeks will be hard. His birthday and Father's Day are coming up and I know the wounds will be opened again.

I know I'm still grieving — grieving that we physically lost him but also that we lost him years ago. A few weeks ago, I was thinking how I always called Dad to ask him how to fix something. Then I realized how long ago it would have been that I would have been able to ask him a question and he would have known the answer. There are days I want to beat the crap out of something, anything, to release this anger. I told my husband to buy me a punching bag for my birthday. He thought I was kidding. I wasn't.

*I still wonder when the day will come that I don't, at some point in the day, have to remind myself that my dad's gone. I don't think anyone understands how much this affects you. — **Cheryl***

♡

When Dad died, on some level it almost seemed like a non-event. That isn't to say I wasn't sad. I was devastated. But, honestly, I'd been grieving him for years. Every time he forgot something — a name or moment we spent together — I grieved. Every time my father looked at me and didn't know who I was, I grieved. Sometimes it felt like the grief, and sadness, would never end. — **Frank**

♡

Mama and I were always very close and I always wondered if I'd be able to live without her. But at the end, she was suffering. I knew she wouldn't want to live like that, she was so sick. It was a blessing when God took her. I never thought I would say something like that. — **Grace**

♡

Currently, I'm relieved she has passed and is no longer suffering. However, I fear I wasn't good enough to her in the last few years. I visited a lot, but not as much as I would have liked and I fear she may have felt abandoned. I regret not being patient enough with her in the early stages. I'm also still very angry my mom suffered with Alzheimer's during the last three years of her life. At times, I resented the woman she had become which made me feel horrible. I would look at her and she wasn't my mom. She sounded like her, but it wasn't her and yet I was stuck with her. I felt selfish and mean for feeling like that, but her grandchildren were robbed of their Nana and I just wanted my best friend back. — **Leslie**

♡

Dad died in 2007 and I have been going to counseling to help me deal with my grief, my denial, my anger. — **Pat**

254 I Love You ... Who Are You?

In my work with hospice, I have had occasion to counsel many people who have lost loved ones. For those people whose parents or spouses had Alzheimer's, I've noticed the grieving process is generally very different.

For them, the grieving process began years ago with the onset of the disease. The mother who used to comfort you has been replaced by someone who is bewildered and trapped in her own confusing world. A father, whose eyes once lit up when he saw you, may no longer remember who you are.

Although the loved one was still alive, a large part of them felt already gone. It's a tremendous loss when the one you love has changed so dramatically. The grieving may have been subtle at first, but it was nevertheless very present. When an Alzheimer's patient dies, many caregivers often tell me, "I started to mourn a long time ago."

They may find themselves not as grief-stricken as others might expect them to be. Some are clearly ready to regain the lives that had been put on hold for years. Other caregivers, however, may continue to grieve for a long, long time.

What is important to remember is that every person, and every relationship, is different. Therefore, how the loss is processed will be unique for each individual. What is completely normal for one person may not be normal for someone else.

Allow grief to take whatever form it needs. Some people may be depressed or angry; others may withdraw or isolate themselves, while others keep as busy as possible. No one can or should tell you what grief should look like because it's an extremely individualized process. Allow grief to take its own course.

Caregiving is a very challenging road. Death means the end of caring for another but hopefully it can mean the beginning of caring for yourself. Take exquisite care of yourself. Honor yourself for what you have done. And may you be richly blessed.

Rev. Cynthia Greb is a hospice chaplain and bereavement counselor.

As you begin putting the pieces of your life back together, you may feel guilty. Caregivers say they remember the first time they laughed or enjoyed themselves after their parent's death and, for an instant, felt terrible guilt.

There will be many "firsts" in the months ahead: the first holiday without your parent, visiting a favorite restaurant for the first time without them, and the first anniversary of their death. Each of these can, to some degree, reopen wounds and bring up emotions for you to deal with. Allow the emotions to come up. Find someone you can talk with; or a way for you to deal with — and move through — the emotions.

Some caregivers had to give themselves permission to go on and enjoy their lives. Realistically, we all know our parent wouldn't want us to spend the remainder of our days grieving for them. But, again, it's a process.

Over time, the level and intensity of your grief, and other emotions, will subside. You'll begin to understand that you can still enjoy your life. You can laugh, you can make plans for the future, and you can put the pieces of your life back together. You *can* go on.

Following the death of your parent, you may feel a numbness, which indicates you are in a place of transition. There is always a period of transition after death — a time when one thing is gone and nothing else has really come to fill its place. Take your time. Let yourself grieve.

After caring for your parent for so long, there is a huge gap that was once occupied by caring for, visiting or thinking about your parent. You may not know what to do with your time or feel lost or empty. This is because the loss has left a hole in your life and in your psyche.

Healing the grief is, quite simply, the process of attending to the "hole" created by the loss of your parent. Fill it with memories, love, and support from others. Know that it takes time. You will begin again. You will begin anew. The only way out is the way through.

You will find that nature hates a void and things will begin to come into your life again. Begin to fill your life with goodness and love. Choose to fill your life with joy. You are stronger, wiser and more aware. You have survived!

Patricia Fares-O'Malley, PhD is a psychologist, educator, international speaker, Bereavement Coordinator for hospice and the author of "Healing The Love Wound."

EPILOGUE

"All is Well": A Mother's Gift

It all began one morning just a few short weeks before my mother's death.

As we neared the final days of Mom's life, every second with her became sacred. Little things like touching her hand or looking into her eyes took on monumental meaning. I held her, sang to her, and stroked her hair. I didn't want to leave her side for fear that, the next time I saw her, she would be gone.

Hospice remained gentle and patient with me through the transition. They continued to explain the physiological changes that were occurring with, and in, my mother. They explained why she no longer wanted to eat or drink. They told me to keep the lights low and the room warm. They also told me the last sense to leave a person was the sense of hearing, so I told Mom repeatedly that I loved her. Even though she remained unresponsive, her eyes closed, I was confident my mother heard me.

Since Mom always loved music, and since it was the holiday season, we kept Christmas carols quietly playing in her room. I made a CD of special music which I played for my mother every morning. It became a special, sacred part of my day with her and, in the weeks that followed, I would learn it was special to my mother, too.

On this morning, like every other morning, my father went in to see my mother first. He kissed her, talked to her and told her he loved her. After he left, Bernice and I went in to see Mom and prepare her for a new day.

As I walked to the side of Mom's bed, I took hold of her hand and prayed for the same miracle I prayed for every morning: the miracle of recognition. Would today be the day Mom magically recognized me and said my name? I desperately wanted to hear my mother speak my name one more time. But like so many days before, Mom stared straight ahead, her eyes vacant and without a hint of recognition.

I kissed Mom, then walked over to turn on the CD. The music on the CD contained several songs by a musician named Karen Drucker. While I had always loved Karen's music, of late, it touched me on an even deeper level. The words to her songs had become particularly poignant and taken on special meaning in these final days with Mom.

I hit the "Play" button and walked back over to help Bernice.

We began to turn Mom on her side so, if necessary, we could change her clothes or the bedding. It was difficult since the pain in Mom's hip was still apparent. She would wince or gasp when we tried to move her. Gratefully, Bernice and I had found a way to move her with as little discomfort as possible. I would slide one hand under Mom's head and another lower down on her body. At the same time, I would say very quietly, "Come here, Mama. Let me hold you." At the sound of my voice, my mother would turn her head, and then her body, towards me.

As Bernice checked Mom and the bedding, I began singing along to the song playing quietly in the background: *"We are connected by the heart...where do you end and where do I start? Anything you pray for...if fear is in your way...I am here to listen, to anything you need to say...Your prayer is my prayer too..."*[1]

Other than an occasional word or sound, Mom was silent. But on that morning, as I held her, Mom stared into my eyes with an intensity I had never seen. She didn't blink or look away. She continued to stare into my eyes, so I stopped singing and held her gaze. I was overcome by an overwhelming feeling of love and tenderness. I could sense that my mother was telling me without words that she loved me. I also knew she was saying goodbye.

When the song ended, I continued to hold her. I kissed her gently. Then, looking back into her eyes, I asked, "Mama, when you get to where you're going, can you just let me know you're okay?" She continued to stare into my eyes, blinked once, then closed her eyes and dozed off.

Several days later, my mother died in the peace and comfort of her home.

Our family decided we wanted something more meaningful than the traditional prayer card for my mother's funeral. I began working on a special memorial booklet about my mother on the night she died. Three days later, the printer called and told me if I wanted the booklet ready in time for Mom's services, he needed the final copy that day.

I hung up the phone, and sat down to turn on my computer. I watched as the hourglass on the computer screen turned over...and over...and over. As I watched it turn, I realized my computer wasn't starting. Had it crashed? And if it had, what was I going to do? Despite constant reminders from my sons to backup my computer, I hadn't. I knew the printer was waiting for the final version. Were we going to have to forego the memorial booklet for Mom's service?

Then music began to play. For an instant, I didn't think anything of it and glanced over at the CD player in my office. It was empty and still turned off.

Confused, I looked back at my computer screen. On it was something which reminded me of the panel on a car radio. I read the words on the panel: *Song In My Soul* and, as I read them, I listened to the music and the words coming out of my computer:

> *"Healed...Whole...Well...Healed...Whole...Well.*
>
> *There is a song in my soul, it sings I am whole. Everywhere I go, it sings I am whole...*
>
> *There is a song in my soul, it sings I am healed. I take a breath and know that I am healed...*
>
> *There is a song in my heart, it sings I am loved. It whispers in my ear, that I am loved.*
>
> *There is a song in my soul, it sings of my joy, it bubbles up from deep inside,*
>
> *Pure, sweet joy.*
>
> *There is a song, it sings I am love. A beaming ray of Spirit's light, I am love.* [2]

I sat at my computer on that quiet December morning, just a few days after my mother's death, and listened to the final refrain of the song: *"I am healed, I am loved, I am joy...All is well. I am well."*[3] As the song ended, the panel and hourglass disappeared and my computer started up.

I sat back, tears streaming down my face. In that instant, I understood — and it all made perfect, beautiful, wonderful sense.

I thought back on the sequence of events that had just occurred and, as I did, any doubt about whether this had been a message from my mother vanished.

First, my mother chose a time when, because of her memorial booklet, I was thinking about, and completely focused on, her.

Then, by not allowing my computer to start, my mother was able to get me to stop long enough to listen to the music that was playing.

By playing the music through my computer, she held my attention because I didn't know *how* to play music on my computer. I played music on the CD player in my office. Had the music played on my CD player, I would have probably thought it was a power surge and went on about my business and not given it a second thought.

Sending her message through music also made sense for many reasons. Music had always been an important part of my mother's life but, after Alzheimer's, music had taken on new meaning. It was a way for our family to continue to connect and communicate with Mom and, in her final days, music had been a sacred part of my day with my mother.

And finally, there was the song itself. It was a song by Karen Drucker — the same woman whose music I had been playing for Mom every morning during our final weeks together. While the song that just played on my computer wasn't on the CD I'd been playing for Mom, it was a song whose words clearly spelled out my mother's message to me — that she was healed, she was fine, and all was well.

A few weeks before Christmas, my mother gave me the gift of knowing.

Knowing that while she had left this earthly plane, my mother was still with me.

Knowing that, in those final days, my mother heard it all: the music, the laughter, the love — and my request for her to let me know she was alright.

Knowing that although it had been years since she had spoken my name or told me she loved me, what my mother's mind had forgotten, her heart never had.

All was well.

APPENDICES

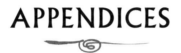

APPENDIX A: RESOURCES

From Our Caregivers & Experts

The following are referenced in this book and/or were created by individuals who shared their experience and expertise in support of this book. Please take a minute to learn more about what they are doing.

Aging Home Health Care
www.aginghomehealthcare.com

Alzheimer's: A Caretaker's Journal
http://mariefostino.blogspot.com

Alzheimer's Art Quilt Initiative
810.637.5586
www.AlzQuilts.org

Care Camp
860.597.0279
www.carecampforkids.com

Humor Matters
714.665.8801
www.humormatters.com

Imagiscape Theater
416.763.6565
www.imagiscape.ca

Kopper Top Life Learning Center-Animal Therapy
336.565.9723
www.koppertop.org

Life Lessons: Coping with Alzheimer's
http://jeannot-lifelessons.blogspot.com/

Living With Alzheimer's
http://whereisannasmind.blogspot.com/

Lost My Mom, Buried My Mind
www.lostmymomburiedmymind.blogspot.com

Puzzles to Remember
www.PuzzlesToRemember.org

Simple Pleasures for Special Seniors
866.278.5300
www.simplepleasuresforspecialseniors.com

The Long Journey
http://c-longhorn.blogspot.com/

Writer Advice
www.writeradvice.com

Alzheimer's & National Organizations

Administration on Aging
202.619.0724
Eldercare Locator: 800.677.1116
www.aoa.gov

Alzheimer's Association
24/7 Helpline: 800.272.3900
Safe Return + MedicAlert:
888.572.8566
www.alz.org

Alzheimer's Disease Education &
Referral Center (ADEAR)
800.438.4380
www.niah.nih.gov/Alzheimers

Alzheimer's Foundation of
America
866.AFA.8484 (866.232.8484)
www.alzfdn.org

Alzheimer's Reading Room
www.alzheimersreadingroom.com

Fischer Center for Alzheimer's
Research Foundation
800.ALZINFO (800.259.4636)
www.alzinfo.org

National Association of Area
Agencies on Aging
202.872.0888
www.n4a.org

National Council on Aging
202.479.1200
www.ncoa.org

U.S. Government — First Gov for
Seniors
800.FEDINFO (800.333.4636)
www.seniors.gov

Caregiver Support and Resources

2-1-1 Information & Referral
Services
www.211.org

A Place for Mom
877.MOMDAD9 (877.666.3239)
www.aplaceformom.com

Caring Bridge
651.452.7940
www.caringbridge.org

Children of Aging Parents
800.227.7294
www.caps4caregivers.org

ElderCare Online
www.ec-online.net

Family Caregiver Alliance
800.445.8106
www.caregiver.org

LotsaHelpingHands
www.lotsahelpinghands.com

National Adult Day Services
Association (NADSA)
877.745.1440
www.nadsa.org

National Alliance for Caregiving
www.caregiving.org

National Association of
Professional Geriatric Care
Managers
520.881.8008
www.caremanager.org

National Caregiving Foundation
800.930.1357
www.caregivingfoundation.org

National Family Caregivers
Association
800.896.3650
www.thefamilycaregiver.org

Next Step In Care
www.nextstepincare.org

Today's Caregiver
www.caregiving.com

Project LifeSaver
877.580.LIFE (877.580.5433)
www.projectlifesaver.org

Financial/Legal Resources

Benefits Check-Up (Service of
National Council on Aging)
www.benefitscheckup.org

Centers for Medicare &
Medicaid Services (CMS)
877.267.2323
www.cms.gov

Medicare
800.MEDICARE (800.633.4227)
www.medicare.gov

National Academy of Elder Law
Attorneys
www.naela.org

National Clearinghouse for Long-
Term Care Information
www.longtermcare.gov

Partnership for Prescription
Assistance
888.4PPANOW (888.477.2669)
www.pparx.org

Paying for Senior Care
641.715.3900, ext. 606151#
www.payingforseniorcare.com

Social Security Administration
800.772.1213
www.ssa.gov

State Health Insurance Assistance
Program (SHIP)
www.shiptalk.org

U.S. Dept. of Veterans Affairs
800.827.1000
www.va.gov

Hospice/End of Life/Grief

Aging with Dignity
888.5WISHES (888.594.7437)
www.agingwithdignity.org

Caring Connections
800.658.8898
www.caringinfo.org

Compassion & Choices
800.247.7421
www.compassionandchoices.org

Hospice Foundation of America
800.854.3402
www.hospicefoundation.org

National Hospice and Palliative Care Organization
800.658.8898
www.nhpco.org

National Hospice Foundation
877.470.6472
www.nationalhospicefoundation.org

Open to Hope
415.994.8263
www.opentohope.com

Products & Supplies

Alzheimer's Store
800.752.3238
www.alzstore.com

Bathing Without a Battle
www.bathingwithoutabattle.unc.edu

Buck and Buck
800.458.0600
www.buckandbuck.com

Caregivers Marketplace
800.888.0889
www.caregiversmarketplace.com

Gold Violin
877.648.8400
www.goldviolin.com

Memory Programs
800.711.7616
www.memoryprograms.com

APPENDIX B:

Finding Support: An Exercise

Begin with two pads of paper. On one pad, draw a line straight down the middle. On the left side of the column, write down the names of everyone you or your parents know. Start with the obvious — immediate and extended family members — brothers, sisters, aunts, uncles, cousins, etc. Next, list names of neighbors, close friends and people you or your parents know from religious or community clubs and organizations. If you know their phone number or e-mail address, jot that down, too.

Don't edit. Don't think "Oh, I could never ask them for help." Just keep writing.

For now, leave the second column blank.

Now, take the second pad of paper and begin to write a list of every way you can think of that someone could help your parent, you or your family now or in the future. Your list might include:

- ❑ driving your parent to a doctor's appointment.
- ❑ phoning or visiting your parent once a week.
- ❑ cooking a meal or picking up take-out.
- ❑ mowing the lawn.
- ❑ weeding the garden.
- ❑ picking up things from the grocery store or drugstore.

You know your circumstances and what will make your days easier and run smoother. Again, just keep writing and when you're done put both pads of paper side-by-side.

As you look at both lists, you'll start to see obvious connections. Perhaps a neighbor goes to the grocery store several times a week and could pick something up for you. Write "grocery store" in the right-hand (blank) column next to their name on the first pad of paper. Or there may be someone from your church who has a landscaping business. Write "mow lawn/weed garden" next to their name.

Continue going through the list until you have put at least one thing in the right-hand column for each person on your first list.

Understand you're not going to pick up the phone and call everyone on the list to tell them what they need to do to help you. This is simply a resource list for you and your family. It is a list of possibilities.

The majority of people really *do* want to help but simply don't know what to do or what you need. Keep this list handy so that, if there is something you need help with, you have a list of people you can contact. When you're stressed, or exhausted, it might be difficult to think clearly and brainstorm who you can reach out to for help. By having this list prepared in advance, it will help assist you in finding at least one person who can help.

This list will also come in handy if one of the individuals (or organizations) on the list contacts you and asks "What can I do to help?" By having this list, you'll be ready to tell them exactly how they can help.

This list is also a valuable resource in the event you (or the primary caregiver) is not available and the person in charge needs to know who to contact for help.

REFERENCES

Chapter Three: The First Steps On Your Journey

[1] Alzheimer's Association, 2008 Alzheimer's Disease Facts and Figures, published in *Alzheimer's & Dementia*, Volume 4, Issue 2.

[2] Alzheimer's Association, 2008 Alzheimer's Disease Facts and Figures, published in *Alzheimer's & Dementia*, Volume 4, Issue 2.

Chapter Four: The Caregiver's Journey

[1] AARP Public Policy Institute (2008, November). *Valuing the Invaluable: The Economic Value of Family Caregiving*, 2008 Update. Washington, DC; Mittelman, M. S., Haley, W., & Roth, D. (2006). *"Improving Caregiver Well-being Delays Nursing Home Placement of Patients with Alzheimer's Disease."* Neurology, 67, 1592-1599.

[2] Alzheimer's Association and National Alliance for Caregiving. *"Families Care: Alzheimer's Caregiving in the United States"*, 2004.

[3] Alzheimer's Association and National Alliance for Caregiving. *"Families Care: Alzheimer's Caregiving in the United States"*, 2004.

[4] MetLife Mature Market Institute. *"The MetLife Study of Alzheimer's Disease: The Caregiving Experience"*, August 2006.

Chapter Five: "All the What Ifs"

[1] *"Perceptions of the Impact of Pet Therapy on Residents/Patients and Staff in Facilities Visited by Therapy Dogs"*. Study conducted by Therapy Dogs International, Inc. www.tdi-dog.org

Chapter Nine: "All Is Well": A Mother's Gift

[1] *"Your Prayer Is My Prayer Too"*, words and music: Karen Drucker. ©TayToones Music BMI 2005 www.karendrucker.com

[2, 3] *"Song In My Soul"*, words: Karen Drucker & Jo Ann Buckner-Rhyne; music: Karen Drucker ©TayToones Music BMI 2005. www.karendrucker.com

INDEX

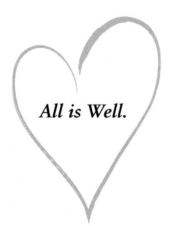

All is Well.

ORDER FORM

Additional copies of this book can be ordered online through the author's website: **www.pattikerr.com** or by mailing this form (along with a check or money order for payment in full) to:

Along the Way Press, PO Box 2443, Flemington, NJ 08822

Please send me _____ copies of *"I LOVE YOU...WHO ARE YOU?: Loving and Caring for a Parent With Alzheimer's."* I have included payment in full (including any applicable sales tax and shipping).

If you would like the book(s) signed, please include that information (be as specific as possible) in the space below:

_____

_____

Shipping information:

Name: _____

Address: _____

City: _____ State: _____ Zip: _____

In the event there are questions regarding your order, please provide the following:

Telephone: _____

Email address: _____

Sales tax: Please add 7% for products shipped to New Jersey addresses.

Shipping within US: $4.95 for Priority Shipping for first book; $2.00 for each additional book

For additional information on orders, shipping, or to arrange to have the author appear for a book signing or speaking engagement for your organization or group, please contact the author directly through her website: www.pattikerr.com

ORDER FORM

Additional copies of this book can be ordered online through the author's website: **www.pattikerr.com** or by mailing this form (along with a check or money order for payment in full) to:

Along the Way Press, PO Box 2443, Flemington, NJ 08822

Please send me _____ copies of *"I LOVE YOU...WHO ARE YOU?: Loving and Caring for a Parent With Alzheimer's."* I have included payment in full (including any applicable sales tax and shipping).

If you would like the book(s) signed, please include that information (be as specific as possible) in the space below:

_____

_____

Shipping information:

Name: _____

Address: _____

City: _____ State: _____ Zip: _____

In the event there are questions regarding your order, please provide the following:

Telephone: _____

Email address: _____

Sales tax: Please add 7% for products shipped to New Jersey addresses.

Shipping within US: $4.95 for Priority Shipping for first book; $2.00 for each additional book

For additional information on orders, shipping, or to arrange to have the author appear for a book signing or speaking engagement for your organization or group, please contact the author directly through her website: www.pattikerr.com